Health Promoting Palliative Care

Health Promoting Palliative Care

Allan Kellehear

Melbourne

OXFORD UNIVERSITY PRESS

Oxford   Auckland   New York

OXFORD UNIVERSITY PRESS AUSTRALIA

Oxford New York
Athens Auckland Bangkok Bogotá
Buenos Aires Calcutta Cape Town Chennai
Dar es Salaam Delhi Florence Hong Kong
Istanbul Karachi Kuala Lumpur Madrid
Melbourne Mexico City Mumbai Nairobi
Paris Port Moresby São Paulo Singapore
Taipei Tokyo Toronto Warsaw

and associated companies in
Berlin Ibadan

OXFORD is a trade mark of Oxford University Press

National Library of Australia
Cataloguing-in-Publication data:

Kellehear, Allan.
    Health promoting palliative care.

    Bibliography.
    Includes index.
    ISBN 0 19 550785 1.

    1. Palliative treatment. 2. Health promotion.
    3. Terminal care. I. Title.

362.175

Edited by Lucy Davison
Indexed by Russell Brooks
Text and cover designed by Cath Lindsey
Typeset by Cath Lindsey
Printed by Kyodo Printing Co. Pte Ltd, Singapore
Published by Oxford University Press,
253 Normanby Road, South Melbourne, Australia

If I had but two loaves of bread, I would sell one and buy hyacinths, for they would feed my soul.

One of several translations of a poem attributed to the
13th century Persian poet Shelkh Muslih-al Din Sadi
(Morris 1958)

Contents

Acknowledgments

The author and publisher are grateful to the following copyright holders for granting permission to reproduce textual material in this book: Australian Council of Social Services for extract from C. Parkinson, *The Self-Help Movement in Australia*, ACOSS, Sydney, 1979; John Smyth for extract from J. Smyth, *A Rationale for Teacher's Pedagogy: A Handbook*, Deakin University Press, Geelong, 1986; Curtis Brown (Australia) for extract from A. Goode (ed.), *More Great Working Dog Stories*, ABC Books, Sydney, 1992; Western Institute of Self Help (WISH) for extract from S. Thorman, *A Journey through Self Help: An Evaluation of Self Help in Western Australia*, WISH, Cottesloe, WA, 1987; and the Palliative Care Unit at La Trobe University for permission to reproduce our 'support group guidelines'.

Every effort has been made to trace the original source of all material reproduced in this book. Where the attempt has been unsuccessful, the authors and publisher would be pleased to hear from the copyright holder concerned to rectify any omission.

Abbreviations

CSMC   Council for the Single Mother and her Child
ESP   extra-sensory perception
EVP   electronic voice phenomena
RCT   randomised control trial
UNICEF   United Nations Children's Fund
WHO   World Health Organization

Preface

These are troubling times for palliative care. Recognition of the importance of palliative care has peaked at a time when governments are attempting to reduce their health care budgets. Today, the desire of policy-makers and practitioners to embrace the holistic ideals of hospice and palliative care comes face-to-face with an ever-diminishing financial capacity to do so. Compromise is in the air. Increasingly, the precious few resources available are being allocated to physical care. Palliative care is frequently mistaken for terminal, end-stage care. It becomes more difficult every day to find evidence that serious resources are being made available to services that take an earlier view and/or a more social or spiritual view of palliative care. At schools or universities, in hospitals or hospices, we are being asked to do more with less. It seems a cruel nonsense to speak about doing more with less. And often it is.

This book offers a series of suggestions that have, at their core, the idea that one might actually do more with more. And the 'more' that can be done is the expansion of the ranks of palliative care by including colleagues and ideas from public health, particularly health promotion. Public health is one area of health care that has enjoyed strong support from governments because of its commonly acknowledged role in 'saving' money. Public health, it is frequently argued, is less expensive than acute and chronic forms of care because its emphasis is on prevention. Notwithstanding the different arguments about the reality of those savings, it is not unreasonable to make the following observation: the ideals of health promotion have much in common with those of palliative care. And the introduction of health promotion into palliative care might greatly renew support for a focus on living with dying that addresses the early stages of dying—the part of palliative care that now seems too difficult for current policy-makers and funding sources.

But there are other reasons to take a close look at the fruitful relationship between health promotion and palliative care. Much has been made of the holistic mission of palliative care—care that is not only physical but also social, psychological, and spiritual. Yet the proliferation of models of what has come to be glibly called 'psychosocial' interventions seems to have little unity and even less theoretical and practical consistency. Social needs are too often conflated with psychological needs. Spiritual issues are frequently subsumed under psychological ones. Clarity, consistency, and definition have been the casualties in a field that gropes for theoretical organisation, for clear guidelines about facilitating health-seeking behaviour at the end of life. Health promotion, on the other hand, is characterised by an abundance of theory and practice about these very issues, but so far it has not met—some say that it shies away from—the field of death, dying, and palliative care. The current troubles in health care demand this state of affairs be brought to an end. This is the central purpose of this book.

In chapter 1 I take the reader through the core concerns of palliative care, identifying what I see as the underdeveloped areas of palliative care practice. The core concerns of health promotion are then outlined, taking care to note common criticism but also to note important overlap with common palliative care interests. The ways that palliative care might usefully combine with health promotion ideas are then outlined, showing what is needed in order for palliative care to be health promoting and what health promotion needs to incorporate to become a valuable source of palliative care.

Chapter 2 is devoted to discussing the goals and practice issues of health promoting palliative care, employing the principles of the Ottawa Charter as a way of organising these topics. I examine possible client groups and program development issues. The manner, stage of illness, and the diversity of social supports relevant to this practice are also discussed. How one might encourage interpersonal reorientation or the reorientation of health services, or combat death-denying health policies and attitudes as part of one's health promoting work, is the focus of the latter parts of the chapter.

Chapters 3–7 are in-depth discussions of the basic principles of health promoting palliative care. Chapter 3 is devoted to an examination of health education theories, processes, and strategies. Chapter 4 is dedicated to an examination of the important topics of death education. Literature pertinent to this area is highlighted for practitioners in this chapter. Chapter 5 is devoted to a general discussion of social supports with a particular focus on support groups in palliative care. The strengths and weaknesses of support groups, the role of these groups in health promotion and palliative care, and a review of some of the practical issues involved are the main concerns of this chapter. Chapter 6 provides an overview of the main areas of interpersonal reorientation for people living with a serious life-threatening illness. We so often discuss health services for people without seriously discussing the experiences of these people. This chapter reviews some of the basic social issues that seriously ill people confront on a daily basis. I attempt to provide readers with a starting point for understanding the nature and extent of the reorientation that these people face, often well before they need hospice care. The final chapter examines the core concerns of environmental and policy development for a health promoting palliative care approach. It outlines strategies for practitioners related to research, education and training, policy change, and private-sector support. The book ends with some final reflections in the conclusion.

I wrote this book primarily for practitioners working alone or in health care institutions. It describes a kind of practice model that can inform the provision of services addressing the social side of serious illness. I believe that this is a promising model for palliative care because it complements the traditional concerns of the field. But this model is also able to offer critical responses to the wider, albeit shrinking, health care systems of today and to their apologetic policies. But you might not agree, in which case this model provides an opportunity to review, and perhaps rethink, your own responses to the policy and practice issues in palliative care that go beyond mere physical care. How might the issues be addressed differently? This question is a good one, and the task and process of exploring it worthwhile and timely.

On the other hand, I am aware that some palliative care practitioners have attempted to incorporate health promotion philosophy into their palliative care practice. I know that some workers are aware of the fruitful connection between the holistic mission of palliative care and the Ottawa Charter. Such practice of health promotion in palliative care, however, has been unusual or uncommon to date, and so often the individual practice has emerged from professional isolation. Theoretical or practical consistency has been a problem. Thus those workers with university connections, for example, have been more able to grapple with research and policy tasks than have those whose funding comes solely from direct service provision. In this way, without a broader debate about what needs to be included or modified in such an approach when used in palliative care, practice can become driven by a politics of convenience rather than by a strived-for vision. The book has been written to open up and provoke this debate, and to encourage a wider interest in developing that vision.

Finally, to some degree, I wrote this book with teaching in mind. Compared with other clinical subjects, so many 'psychosocial' programs or models in palliative care seem to have no underlying philosophy or theory. Who can blame students of palliative care who might mistakenly believe that these kinds of interventions or approaches are so arbitrary that anyone can simply invent them? It is crucial to know that the social care of others can be systematic and, therefore, thorough in its attention and concerns. The social expression of compassion should not be idiosyncratic; its analysis should not be impressionistic. The delivery of effective professional care always arises from planned and organised models that are both philosophically sound and sensitive to the everyday realities of people's experience.

These are values that are shared by a number of personal friends who have been influential in my thinking and who provided critical feedback on an earlier draft of this book. In this respect, I would like to thank Derek Colquhoun (Health Promotion, Ballarat University), a long-time friend and collaborator, who took time to talk with me about the ideas in the book, suggest readings, and discuss the earlier draft. Derek's own research and writing on 'health promoting schools' has been important in shaping my interest in health promotion.

I am also grateful for the usual feedback I have received from Jan Fook (Social Work, Deakin University). Jan is special to me for several reasons: because of her personal influence as a prominent writer and theorist of social work practice; because she reads all my manuscripts with great care and patience; but mainly because, as my companion in life, she has been unwavering in her commitment to encouraging and supporting my interest in death and dying topics when many thought, and still think, it an odd interest for a sociologist to pursue.

Several other people played important roles in providing feedback, information, or support in the writing of this book. Jeanne Daly (Public Health, La Trobe University) has encouraged my ideas in this area almost since I began developing them some time ago when I was working briefly in the alcohol and drug public-health area. Additionally, I thank her for her good humour in allowing me to reproduce, in one of the later chapters of this book, one of her holiday postcards to me.

Mary Fraser (Sociology, La Trobe University, Bendigo) has encouraged me to maintain and employ my affection for classical literature. Gene James (Philosophy, University of Memphis) provided feedback on the philosophical dimensions of the ideas underpinning health promoting palliative care. Greg Barton (Religious Studies, Deakin University), Abdullah Saeed (Asian Studies, University of Melbourne), and Joel Nathan (Palliative Care Unit, La Trobe University)—the most adept Internet 'surfer' I have ever met—assisted in what turned out to be a major hunt for the author of the Sufi quotation that opens the book. I thank all of these colleagues for their own special contribution to the style and content of this work.

The foundation staff at the Palliative Care Unit at La Trobe University have been great supporters of the philosophy of health promoting palliative care and, since our coming together, great friends and colleagues too. The book has also been revised and polished in the light of their considerable advice and experience in the area. I would like to thank the members of that team: Gail Bateman, Valerie Cotronei, Joel Nathan, and Bruce Rumbold. In particular, Bruce Rumbold has been a dedicated and careful reviewer of my ideas, and there is no doubt that the final product has particularly benefited from his critical eye.

I would also like to thank two other people who have played different but important roles in the support and development of the ideas in this book. These two people have been crucial in helping me to establish the health promoting palliative care unit at La Trobe University—a development that reinforced my belief in the value of the main ideas in this book. In this regard, I extend my public gratitude to Professor Stephen Duckett, Dean of Health Sciences at La Trobe University, and the Hon. Rob Knowles, Minister for Health and Aged Care for the state of Victoria, for their active, personal interest in these ideas. They may not agree with all of the ideas in this book. Above and beyond these differences, however, we have together been able to find and share some common vision of how things could be improved in palliative care.

Finally, I dedicate this book to the memory of Matsui 'I'm-sorry-no-hair' Shinjiro—an exceptionally dear and kind member of my family who welcomed the unwelcome, saw with his hands, and spoke through clocks. As the ancients used to say of their beloved fallen: 'may the earth lie lightly upon thee'.

Allan Kellehear
Geelong West
June 1998

1

Introducing Health Promotion to Palliative Care

> . . . we have to learn a new way of seeing.
>
> Or an old way we have forgotten how to use.
>
> *Reanney 1994, p. 1*

On the last page of the last chapter of the *Oxford Textbook of Palliative Medicine*, Jan Stjernsward (in Doyle et al. 1993, p. 814) argues for the need to adopt a 'rational approach' to palliative care. He stresses the importance of taking a public health, rather than simply an institution-alised, approach. Tantalising though these final words are, Stjernsward provides us with few clues about what this might involve beyond a few educational strategies. In this book, and particularly in this first chapter, my aim is to introduce readers to one promising public health model of palliative care for the future: a health promotion model.

The terms 'palliative care' and 'health promotion' seem to be contra-dictory, almost by definition. Palliative care is care for those people whose health has so failed them that they are considered to be entering their 'final illness'. Health promotion is assumed to be for the well, so that they might stay that way. The conventional approach to health pro-motion has highlighted illness prevention. The conventional approach to palliative care has emphasised illness management. However, it is unnecessary to distinguish so sharply between the two, and in this chapter, I will examine and evaluate the usefulness of both of these views.

Palliative care principles can and should be extended in valuable ways towards the ideas of health promotion. At the same time, it is fair to observe that health promotion has marketed itself as a death–deny-ing activity, ignoring the health needs of dying people as though they had no such needs.

In the first part of this chapter, I will reflect on the conventional meaning of palliative care and identify what I see as its current limita-tions. I will attempt to trace the possibilities for health promotion from some of the core, but so far underdeveloped, elements of palliative care. In the second section of the chapter, I will introduce the central ideas of health promotion, summarising its basic aims and competencies, and outlining some of its key problems.

From these comparisons and contexts, I will then describe what health promotion might look like in the context of palliative care. The final purpose of my introduction to health promoting palliative care is to identify and discuss these new principles.

CORE CONCERNS OF PALLIATIVE CARE

There are several features of palliative care on which most observers can agree. Palliative care is a multi-professional form of health care designed to care for the person with a life-threatening, although more usually terminal, illness. This care is meant to be holistic, meaning that it is designed to attend not just to the physical needs of the dying person, but also to the psychological, social, and spiritual needs as well. The aims of the care are to relieve distress and to alleviate the symptoms of a progressive illness that is no longer responsive to medical curative treatment.

The World Health Organization (WHO) (1990; see also Johnston & Abraham 1995) asserts that there are several basic principles underlying good palliative care. Good palliative care:

- neither hastens nor postpones death
- relieves distress
- integrates the psychological with the spiritual dimensions of life
- provides appropriate support for the dying person and his or her family.

These principles echo remarks by Cicely Saunders (1987, p. 57), who recognises palliative care as the 'control of distress' rather than the 'treatment for cure'. Although Saunders recognises that most palliative care occurs at the end of life, in the last few days or weeks, she argues that palliative care should also apply across the span of the disease from the time of diagnosis.

Saunders and many other writers (see Clark 1994) also recognise and emphasise the multidimensional nature of care: physical, psychological, social, and spiritual. The British National Council for Hospice and Specialist Palliative Care Services (1995) also recognises these core aspects of palliative care, arguing for its multi-professional, across-the-disease, non-curative nature. As Deborah Dudgeon and her colleagues (1995) have observed, palliative care is about quality of life, not quantity.

We can thus summarise the core theoretical aspects of palliative care in the following way:

> Palliative care is:
> - mainly for patients with terminal illness
> - multi-professional
> - physical, emotional, social, and spiritual care
> - aimed at relieving distress (symptoms not disease)
> - applicable across the span of the disease

A closer examination of these core aspects of palliative care shows us that they are, on every count, aspects that are either contested or unrepresentative of the form of palliative care currently being delivered in many places.

Let us begin with the idea of multi-professionalism. Not all observers or practitioners of palliative care view its practice in such magnanimous and interdisciplinary terms. Patty Hodder and Anne Turley (1989, p. 2), for example, view palliative care as 'one of the newest and most rapidly developing medical disciplines'. Other professionals, they assert, are involved in palliative care as 'other services' or as 'components' of the palliative care service system. Neil MacDonald (1993) is less certain about the exclusive medical nature of palliative care than are Hodder and Turley, but nevertheless argues that palliative care is simply care based on 'good medical practice' (p. 65).

The British National Council for Hospice and Specialist Palliative Care Services (1995), in an effort to be as inclusive as possible in its view of multi-professionalism, actually lists the professions that it sees as the main contributors to this style of care: social and welfare workers, doctors, psychologists, psychiatrists, counsellors and family therapists, dietitians, nurses, occupational and diversional therapists, clergy, volunteers, and complementary therapists. Notably missing from this list are social science and public-health workers, a range of non-clinical staff who are not immediately identified with an institutional model of care. How important or significant might omitting the perspectives of these approaches be?

The significance of these omissions only becomes clear when one examines the next core aspect of palliative care: the purportedly multidimensional nature of its care. Palliative care should address itself not merely to the physical problems of the dying person but also to the person's psychological, social, and spiritual needs. The regularity with which we see the 'social' almost imperceptibly drop out of discussions about palliative care is significant. The way in which psychosocial issues soon become more 'psycho-' than social is also notable.

M. Kearney (1992), for example—in an article pleading for palliative care not to sell itself short by confining its gaze to physical symptoms—confines his idea of 'beyond the physical' to the psychological dimensions of subjective experience and emotion. He reiterates the need for palliative care to be multidimensional and argues for the need to attend carefully to the physical *and* emotional *and* spiritual. The social does not receive a mention, or is perhaps subsumed under 'emotional' or 'spiritual'. Note also that when Gail Johnston and Charles Abraham (1995) discuss the WHO guidelines themselves, they too omit the term 'social', emphasising instead the need to integrate the psychological with the spiritual. However, they appear merely to be repeating the omission of the original WHO discussion.

The social-support literature in palliative care might be expected to give social life greater prominence, or at least provide greater detail on it. But this has not always been the case either. Johnston and Abraham (1995), for example, discuss the 'support system' of the dying person, by which they simply mean the communication and awareness issues in terminal care. MacDonald (1993) acknowledges the importance of 'psychosocial issues' when discussing priorities in education and research in palliative care, but spends his entire article discussing symptom control.

Eileen Chiverton (1997) sees social support in terms of care behaviour: helping communication, the 'regulation and management of feeling', and problem-solving. Gunn Grande and colleagues (1997) narrow the definition of support by using even more specific characteristics, such as transport, personal care, housework, communication, and kindness. It is only when we look at palliative care in the HIV/AIDS area that the literature begins to acknowledge aspects of social care that relate to actual interpersonal issues. These aspects go beyond the narrow confines of 'care behaviour' but are nevertheless relevant to it.

Frank Foley and colleagues (1995) identify a collection of these concerns as they apply to people with HIV/AIDS: peer support, sexuality, substance use and abuse, family dynamics, multiple losses, social norms and stigma, and the absence of social rituals for life transitions. Foley and his colleagues (1995, p. 19) present a number of experiences that are offered to readers as 'challenging the palliative paradigm'.

The absence of social science and public health perspectives and input is palpable in palliative care literature and practice. This has led to one dimension—social aspects of care—being underdeveloped, despite the genuine desire to address these concerns. Often, social issues are subsumed under the category of 'psychosocial' issues, where this category is used. Once categorised in this way, social issues are linked strongly with psychological experiences and problems.

Although social issues and problems often manifest as individual worries, they are not any more psychological because of that. Sometimes interpersonal issues must be addressed interpersonally. Only so much can be achieved by attitude change and rationalisation. Sometimes groups of people need to come together. Sometimes they need to be kept apart. And sometimes, people need to learn new ways of relating to others once their usual roles and expectations have altered.

The third core meaning of palliative care—the idea that this form of care is about relieving the distress of symptoms, about improving the quality and not the quantity of life—has also created differences of opinion. Kearney (1992) recognises that curing as well as caring can also take place as part of palliative care. Although uncommon, cure is an idea that should not be seen as totally foreign because palliative care also pursues, at the very least, the cure of certain troublesome symptoms.

From the HIV/AIDS area once again, Foley and his colleagues (1995) remind us that with HIV/AIDS the conventional distinctions between active treatment and palliative intent are not always clear and, at the very least, may be blurred and coexistent. In this way, the central and exclusive meaning of palliative care as a form of palliation must give way to the possibility that active treatment is not necessarily excluded. How well and how much we understand these issues depend on the type and stage of the disease we are confronting. Palliative care is not, therefore, always for those with terminal illness alone, but more broadly, it is for those whose disease presents a significant and increasing threat to life.

Perhaps a more useful way of addressing this problematic aspect of palliative care is to understand the issue in terms of priorities. The main priority in palliative care is to relieve distress rather than to pursue active treatment, especially when every indication suggests that active treatment will be to no avail. On the other hand, treatment that might extend and improve the life of someone who has a life-threatening illness is obviously not precluded, keeping in mind that in some cases, such as in HIV/AIDS, such treatment might be pursued quite actively.

Finally, although the principle of palliative care across the course of the disease is recognised, in practice this principle seems to be largely ignored (as noted by Saunders 1987; and Dudgeon et al. 1995). Dudgeon and colleagues compared seventy-five terminal-phase patients with an equal number of first-reoccurrence cancer patients and found that the major difference between the two groups related to the severity of physical distress. If the psychosocial issues are to be taken seriously, then there appeared to be no significant differences between the groups in terms of their psychosocial needs. Dudgeon and colleagues use this observation to argue for earlier palliative care services for the seriously life-threatened ill.

In summary then, we are able to identify five areas of the core aspects of palliative care that seem underdeveloped.

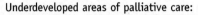

Underdeveloped areas of palliative care:
- social science and public health perspectives
- the social side of care
- early-stage care (not just end-stage)
- active treatment of disease
- care for those with life-threatening illness (not simply terminal)

Although there has been no shortage of comment about these problems, especially the emphasis on terminal end-stage care, there have been few suggestions about how to address them. A strong alternative framework that can address these issues in an organised way has not eventuated. On the other hand, developments in public health, and especially in health promotion, are able to offer suggestions regarding a way forward.

The palliative care ideas themselves suggest the basis on which to extend palliative care ideas and practices to incorporate those from health promotion. There is a need to address, in more specific and concrete ways, the social concerns and problems of the dying. There is especially a need to address these concerns where they have a significant impact on the health and comfort of those with serious illness. We have learnt from the HIV/AIDS area that activities to maintain good health and extend life span have a legitimate place in good palliative care practice. And finally, many practitioners are now acknowledging that much useful work with seriously ill people might be done earlier, rather than later, in the course of their illnesses. This is particularly true with regard to psychological, social, and spiritual issues, regardless of how these are defined. Some of the core concerns of health promotion suggest useful ways to address these development issues in palliative care. We will review these core concerns in the next part of this chapter.

CORE CONCERNS OF HEALTH PROMOTION

Health promotion is not a complicated idea. Basically it is any combination of strategies that are designed to improve people's health. Most of the time, this involves a combination of education, information, and service delivery (Sindall 1992). Health promotion is one part of a broader approach to public health, which includes ideas such as health protection (laws and regulations), preventive medicine, health education and policy, and community action.

Mary Louise O'Connor and Elizabeth Parker (1995) argue that, historically, health promotion has expressed itself in one of three ways:

1 a conventional medical approach (for instance, through immunisation or screening campaigns)
2 a behavioural approach (for instance, by paying attention to risk factors such as smoking, poor diets, accident prevention, and so on
3 social-environmental approaches (for example, through scrutiny of, and policy development regarding, workplaces, housing, or transport issues)

But mostly these days, health promotion aspires to a more integrated approach, viewing health not as some idiosyncratic phenomenon but rather as part of a wider pattern of life. True, health has biological (that is, genetic) determinants, but health is also largely socially determined. Patterns of health and illness reflect patterns of work and play, the quality and style of a person's relationships, and the advantages and drawbacks of their age, gender, culture, and social class situations. Ilona Kickbush (1989) argues that the pattern of one's life is inextricably bound together in these ways. A narrow focus on behaviour alone—separated from other life contexts, meanings, pressures, and supports—makes little sense. In that way, for example, buckling one's seatbelt has everything to do with conformism, one's self-concept or identity as a citizen, simple fear of fines, personal habits, car designs, national laws, *and* being personally motivated. Kickbush argues that minor relationships—both in terms of health care and self-care—emerge as part of that greater pattern.

Ideas such as Kickbush's have led to the development and subsequent adoption of the WHO policy on health promotion. This was enshrined in the Ottawa Charter in 1986, and subsequently ratified in the Jakarta Statement in 1997. Most texts on health promotion make the Ottawa Charter central to their discussions, and many other texts that argue for the establishment of 'health promoting' settings (such as schools, workplaces, or hospitals) apply the Ottawa Charter principles to those settings. The Ottawa Charter includes five major 'action' statements.

> The Ottawa Charter for Health Promotion
> 1 Build public policies that support health.
> 2 Create supportive environments.
> 3 Strengthen community action.
> 4 Develop personal skills.
> 5 Reorient health services.

The first principle asserts the need to identify obstacles to health and to develop policies to remove them so that making 'healthy choices' will be an easier task for everyone. The second principle alerts us to the need to make all environments—work, leisure, and health care settings—conducive to health. More specifically, the term 'environment' here might also apply to cultural, situational, physical, temporal, and life experiences (Stokols 1992). The third principle encourages us to strengthen community action. The central message here is to emphasise that health care should be *participatory*. Professional work must be work *with,* rather than *on,* others. It is important to recognise that social relationships are important for coping with stress and maintaining health. In that context, it is crucial that supports and networks should be strengthened to complement other health care activities. The fourth principle promotes the development of personal skills. Information and education about health should be provided so that people can learn about, prepare for, and cope with health maintenance and illness experiences. Finally, the last principle advises that health services should be reoriented. The values of participation, mediation, advocacy, and enabling should not be confined to health professionals and the health sector but should extend to other sectors of society. Health promotion should be intersectoral and involve many groups and professions. Health promotion, like public health itself, is for *all* people, not just certain sections of the community.

The core concerns that emerge from a perusal of contemporary health promotion literature, then, are: the participatory nature of health activity; the importance of recognising the social character of health; the value of education and information; the importance of intervening during times of wellness as well as during illness; and the broad responsibility for promoting health, involving individuals, families, communities, and governments.

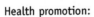

Health promotion:
- is participatory
- recognises the social character of health and illness
- emphasises education, information, and policy development
- is designed for the well and the ill
- is everyone's responsibility, not just the individual's

A number of people have identified problems with this view of health promotion. Bunton and others (1995) provide the best overview of these misgivings. Most of this criticism derives from critical social science perspectives, particularly from feminist and anti-racist quarters. There are four major points.

First, despite rhetoric to the contrary, much health promotion is concentrated on individual help and tends to neglect broader environmental and policy initiatives.

Second, interpersonal interventions and advice, such as they are, are sometimes naive. Admonitions and health advice aimed at changing people's behaviour have not always taken into full account the fact that some people do not have sufficient interpersonal power or social resources to participate or comply. Sexual advice to women, for example, must consider the possible problems of gender inequality in some relationships.

Third, the idea of participation has not always included minority groups, and when they have been included, this has sometimes been passive inclusion. In this way, members of minority groups may be receivers of 'education and information', but since representatives of those groups were not part of the original service design, some of the advice will be culturally inappropriate or difficult for them to act upon.

Finally, health promotion messages have been accused of reinforcing stereotypes and social inequalities in society. Sarah Nettleton and Robin Bunton (1995, p. 45) provide the example of an advertising campaign aimed at encouraging teenagers to think about their automobile-driving habits. Health promotion advertisements remind teenagers that accidents could lead to disablement, which would curtail their enjoyment of a healthy life. A wheelchair is the key image used to signal that warning. This image reinforces community notions of deviance and marginality by supporting and reproducing the idea that people in wheelchairs are somehow less able to enjoy a 'full' life. The message is that health and enjoyment of life are incompatible with serious disablement. Within the community, these kinds of messages are sources of the stigma associated with disablement and challenge the idea that social equality can be achieved by anyone other than the able-bodied.

What is more, this kind of message also undermines the fundamental idea that health is a social experience of well-being by returning to the simplistic and older notion of health as absence of illness and disablement. This is not a definition of health that is compatible with the current ideals of health promotion.

Problems of health promotion:
- environmental and policy initiatives that are underdeveloped
- naive interpersonal interventions
- non-inclusive participation
- cultural reproduction

In addition to the implications that these problems might have for health promotion programs generally, these problems have a particular relevance to issues of death, dying, and palliative care.

The terminally ill are a key group consistently omitted from the health promotion discourse. Occasionally, those with a life-threatening illness, such as people with HIV/AIDS, are included in this discourse, but those with terminal cancer, for example, are given little attention. In this way, health promotion once again retreats to the older, simpler, and mechanistic notions of health as the absence of illness rather than the now widely accepted idea of health as a situation in which a sense of well-being is maximised.

Seriously ill people can, and should have, periods of positive well-being, and as a community, we should be enhancing those times. However, such ideas do not feature in current health promotion texts. The even older, and equally negative, idea that the seriously ill are 'beyond hope' and that they represent 'failure' to health professionals is suggested by this rather telling silence within the health promotion literature. Just as palliative care might be more positive in its aims— promoting health rather than simply ameliorating distress—health promotion might be less death-avoiding, and might take an interest in the health and well-being of those whose current illness just happens to be incurable.

Why should the prospect of death, an event more certain than illness, exclude anyone from health promotion consideration? Why should there be an inverse relationship between prognosis of a terminal disease and interest from public health workers? Do health professionals need to learn all over again that dying does not, and should not, disqualify anyone from quality health and social care? Seriously ill people still qualify as members of the 'public', and so the offerings of public health, including the promise and support of health promotion, are legitimately theirs also. Maintaining a healthy body, mind, and spirit, for example, can be crucial to warding off infections that might threaten and erode the immune system of someone with HIV. Accepting medical and complementary treatments during the course of cancer or cardiac failure, no matter how serious the stage, may help prolong life, improve its experienced quality, and/or help a person to cope with the side-effects of treatment. Since one of the greatest fears of those with a life-threatening illness is the prospect of loss of control over their health and their lives more generally, health promotion can be an important source of empowerment and support. Information can challenge personal fears and change attitudes. Participation can renew confidence and a sense of agency. Support can encourage hope and be a valuable and steady source of comfort.

Health promotion can also play a role in improving the quality of life in times of disease remission. And, of course, the jury is still out on the causes of apparent spontaneous and permanent remissions. Some people will pursue that particular hope wherever it might lead them. Health promotion might provide a measure of critical guidance to these people, offering some advocacy and protection from the perils of charlatans and extortionists. Undoubtedly, health promotion has an important role to play for those with life-threatening and terminal illnesses.

Finally then, the only real question that remains is: what would health promotion look like for those whose illness is likely to end in death? In other words, what might the core concerns of a health promoting palliative care be?

CORE CONCERNS OF A HEALTH PROMOTING PALLIATIVE CARE

When you compare the core concerns of palliative care with those of health promotion, it is relatively simple to see the lessons that each may provide for the other. Both palliative care and health promotion have underdeveloped areas that, if each approach were to study the other's mission seriously, might usefully be redressed. Workers in palliative care might quickly see that adopting some of health promotion's core concerns would provide the social science and public health perspectives that palliative care sorely needs. And health promotion perspectives are not simply policy perspectives or perspectives designed for change on a large-scale, organisational level. There is much in health promotion that is oriented towards work with individuals, and in this sense health promotion has much to offer the mainly individual-oriented practice of palliative care.

Because ideas about what constitutes 'social' care in the palliative context are often underdeveloped, the ideas of health promotion are a ready source of sociological and political detail about particular areas of social life that might be pertinent to the health of everyone, including those with life-threatening illnesses.

Because early-stage care is underdeveloped in palliative care, the early-stage emphasis of health promotion will also offer many useful suggestions for the practice of health promoting palliative care. Health promotion has always emphasised health management rather than illness management, and so its strategies are designed principally, though not exclusively, for times of wellness. These are times that are also experienced by many people with early-stage terminal or life-threatening illnesses.

The palliative principle that active treatment is not always incompatible with life-threatening illness begs the question of what kind of treatment interventions might be possible for most people with such illnesses, many of whom will also be undergoing palliative medical interventions of one sort or another. The education and information emphasis of health promotion can play an important and complementary role in any such traditional treatments of the seriously ill. For both patients and treating professionals, an educational and information emphasis is an unobtrusive strategy for health promotion. However, in recognising the value of education and information, one should also recognise that diverse reactions and decisions among patients are possible, even likely. Some of these changes may alter, or even reverse, the expectations and decisions that people have had or have made about conventional treatments.

Finally, health promotion provides palliative care with the theoretical impetus for a more participatory and structural approach to health care. It is the desire of many palliative care professionals to increase the control that seriously ill people exercise in relation to their disease, and a health promotion approach can only further enhance such a goal. The idea that professionals 'know best' may be further challenged by the experience of the seriously ill, particularly if earlier education and information programs encourage them to become actively involved in their own care. Once again, we must recognise that, in some cases, this may involve a conscious decision on the part of some people to surrender themselves to a traditional, dependent 'sick role'. Some people may not favour a participatory style of health care.

The 'structural' approach of health promotion—that is, the serious attention paid to policy development and the wider context of health care—might also be adopted as a welcome aspect of palliative care. A health promoting palliative care might usefully seek a policy role in broader public-health developments that actively seek to reduce the idea that death and dying are marginal experiences. Such developments might combat the unhelpful idea that serious illness occurs when health and health care have failed. The idea that palliative care settings might also be more than interventionist clinical settings—that they might be positively health promoting—is also a challenge that is suggested by a structural approach to palliative care.

There is also much that palliative care can offer to contemporary health promotion. For one thing, seriously ill people ought to be seen as qualifying for health promoting attention. Dying is not the opposite of health; death is. And dying people, contrary to some beliefs, are not dead. People who are 'dying'—that is, those who live with a terminal or life-threatening illness—are simply people with *chronic* illness who often know that they will die in a short while. Viewing it in a philosophical way, the terminally ill are forced to confront what—despite our fantasies of day-to-day invulnerability—is real for all of us. Any health promotion strategy that does not admit this insight into its policy ruminations is death-denying. Rather than promoting well-being, this lack of acknowledgment returns us, once again, to antique notions of health.

Logically following from this recognition that terminal and life-threatening illnesses have a legitimate place in health promotion is the idea that health promotion at the end of life is a valid concept and a valuable practice. Clearly, the traditional blindness of health promotion to this argument parallels palliative care's neglect of the opposite end of the illness trajectory. But while palliative care may not have given enough practical attention to the earlier stage of terminal illness, it has always openly recognised its importance. Health promotion, on the other hand, has only served the terminally ill if those people have become part of a 'chronic illness' program. The fact that such participants might die soon has done little to alter the offerings of these programs. For this particular population of people, then, health promotion programs have offered less than they might have.

Health promotion, like palliative care, has recognised the 'multidimensional' aspects of health and has emphasised the physical, emotional, and social aspects of health. Palliative care has gone one better.

Palliative care has also identified spiritual care as integral to people's well-being. I will not go into the debates about definitions of the term 'spiritual' here—debates not that dissimilar, after all, to those about terms such as 'physical', 'social', and 'psychological'. It is sufficient to note that, whether we define 'spiritual' as religious, existential, or philosophical dimensions of life, its presence and possible importance has been overlooked by health promotion. It is timely and important to remedy this omission.

Finally, death needs to be considered in relation to Kickbush's 'greater pattern' of life concerns and within contexts that are relevant to health. What death might mean—and, more particularly, what death might mean to people at different times and places in their lives—can have an important bearing on what they might expect from health and from health promotion. Although some people may expect health promotion to be death-denying, a good many people, I expect, will not share that view. Others may want support to develop a realistic, dignified, and prepared response to the occasion when life chooses to leave them.

Given these complementary correspondences in emphasis and development, what might the goals of a health promoting palliative care look like?

1 Health promoting palliative care should be about providing education and information for health, dying, and death. It might perform this function with people who live with a life-threatening or terminal illness by providing not only health education but also death education.

2 Health promoting palliative care should provide social supports, especially personal and community supports. In other words, support groups might play an important role in this form of health care, but so too will coordinating wider support services that are not normally associated with health—for example, solicitors or funeral professionals.

3   Health promoting palliative care should also encourage interpersonal problem-solving, where this is relevant. Those with terminal or life-threatening conditions need sometimes to be prepared for personal changes so that social skills are developed to cope with those changes. Problems, where these are perceived as problems, might be shared with others in the same predicament.

Finally, there needs to be some formal environmental and policy development in traditional palliative care to enhance the health promoting image and offerings of all palliative care services. Such development has two goals:

4   encouraging a reorientation of traditional palliative care services to see the benefits of a health promoting approach
5   combating death–denying health policies and attitudes in the wider society

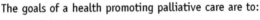

> The goals of a health promoting palliative care are to:
> - provide education and information for health, dying, and death
> - provide social supports—both personal and community
> - encourage interpersonal reorientation
> - encourage reorientation of palliative care services
> - combat death-denying health policies and attitudes

The goals of health promoting palliative care are consistent with the Ottawa Charter, discussed earlier in this chapter. The aims of health promoting palliative care encourage the building of public policies that support health for those who live with terminal or life-threatening illness; they encourage the creation of supportive environments, strengthen community action and personal skills, and encourage the reorientation of health services, particularly those providing palliative care.

How might these goals be achieved? Providing health education for health, dying, and death means providing tailored health education programs that include areas related to diet, alternative therapy, alternative or second medical opinions and advice, and information about the type and nature of a person's illness and the treatment effects. This kind of information can help give people a sense of control and support.

But a health education relevant to those who live with the threat of death is also one that incorporates death education. Death education can serve similar functions to the usual health education programs: providing a forum for the dissemination and discussion of death-related issues—such as social preparations for death, philosophical, existential, or religious (that is, spiritual) discussions about death, or information and education about grief and loss.

Social supports can be provided through support groups, through interpersonal skills training, and by networking the different agencies that are relevant to the needs of those with life-threatening illnesses—legal interests, funeral interests, complementary therapists, the churches, and many other related service areas. Coordinating or introducing these relationships may strengthen the potential for community support for these people in ways previously not brought together.

Interpersonal reorientation may be achieved by offering interpersonal skills support derived from evidence-based information about the problems that people with certain life-threatening illnesses encounter. The creation and use of the support groups and/or self-help groups mentioned above can also play an important role here. Problem-solving and sharing among people in the same or similar situation can provide a participatory and less professionalised source of interpersonal learning. People are able to view their problems simply as social problems that they can solve themselves rather than private problems that may call for a 'professional' or 'therapeutic' response.

Palliative care services must be reoriented if health promotion is to be seen as not just the preserve of those in 'early-stage' illness, or those privileged enough to live in the bigger cities, where, some might believe, the better hospitals, specialists, or health technologies exist. Health promoting palliative care should be offered by all palliative care services.

Combating death–denying health policies is an important and crucial task if the marginal stereotype and experience of those with life-threatening and terminal illness is to be confronted—and opposed. There should also be strategies to develop a greater awareness of death and of the need to support people with life-threatening illnesses in the wider society—through media campaigns, peak public health bodies, and tertiary education and training strategies. In other words, the reorientation of palliative care services and the combating of death-denying health policies require environmental and policy development.

Core concerns of health promoting palliative care:
- health education
- death education
- social supports
- interpersonal reorientation
- environmental and policy development

WHAT HEALTH PROMOTING PALLIATIVE CARE IS NOT

Some practitioners might argue that many traditional palliative care services already offer social supports, health education, or 'counselling' and are therefore very much 'health promoting' services at present. There are several points to be made with respect to such claims.

First, a health promoting palliative care is not an approach to care that simply incorporates and displays one, two, or even three of the core concerns of this approach. Supplying health education or social supports does not make a palliative care service health promoting any more than the provision of pain relief and a chaplain constitutes a conventional palliative care service. The practice of health promoting palliative care is a practice that embraces *all* the concerns together, in concert.

Second, the particular strengths of health promoting palliative care are in its social emphasis, its special relevance to the early stages of illness, and its concern with changing community attitudes and general health policies. The 'social' emphasis means that people are encouraged to identify their own needs, direct their own self-help, and seek to engage with others in similar situations to themselves. Health promoting palliative care is participatory. Traditional counselling of the psychodynamic variety has little to do with this approach.

Because of its particular concern with the early stage of an illness, many of the people involved in health promoting palliative care may not necessarily be targeted by conventional palliative care services unless those services adopt a deliberate policy of soliciting them. In resource terms, the desire to reach this client group could still run into difficulties. Many palliative care services, for instance, may effectively be prevented from working with this client group because the government-established criteria for who is eligible for these kinds of services are often too restrictive. The criterion for eligibility is often a patient life expectancy of less than six or three months. Today's palliative care services may need to broaden their reach to service people who have recent diagnoses of life-threatening illnesses.

Finally, the concern with policy development and health promoting palliative care environments means that palliative care services must attempt to become part—and a seriously acknowledged part—of public health policies, as well as their professional and research activities. Health promoting palliative care is not an additional 'thing to do'. More fundamentally, health promoting palliative care is about shifting our practice approach and philosophy.

In the next chapter, I will revisit the goals of health promoting palliative care and identify and examine the important practice issues that need to be considered if those goals are to be achieved satisfactorily.

I will discuss target populations, assessment and program development issues, and issues of control and authority, and I will revisit the criticisms of health promotion programs as these might apply in health promoting palliative care services.

2

Goals and Practice Principles

Un cabello haze sombra

The least hair makes a shadow

Spanish proverb

To whom is health promoting palliative care aimed? How and when should it be practised, and why? What are the program-development issues for institutions, or for individual practitioners? How can one successfully juggle and achieve the different goals and demands of a health promoting palliative care? These and other questions go to the heart of the practice of the health promoting palliative care model.

I divide this chapter into sections that address and discuss each of the goals of health promoting palliative care. My aim is to describe the central practice principles of a health promoting palliative care with an eye to meeting its main goals. During the discussion, I provide examples and suggestions that might illustrate the philosophy of the model beyond mere theoretical discussion of it.

The goals to be discussed are:

1 the provision of education and information for health, dying, and death
2 the provision of social supports, both personal and community
3 the encouragement of interpersonal reorientation
4 the reorientation of palliative care services
5 the combating of death-denying health policies and attitudes

The final section of the chapter will discuss other development issues in the practice model—for example, how individuals or institutions offering such programs will develop minor variations of the model. The importance of the development of *all* core concerns will be discussed alongside problems that have been associated with traditional health promotion.

PROVIDING EDUCATION AND INFORMATION FOR HEALTH, DYING, AND DEATH

To whom?

The answer to this question is simple: anyone who thinks they might die soon. For palliative care services, this will consist mainly of people who live with a life-threatening or terminal illness. But, more broadly, health promoting palliative care is, or should be, relevant to anyone who seriously believes that they might die soon. Among these possible clients are all older people. These might be people in the second half of their lives who feel that they might benefit from special health information and education about their particular age group. They might also feel that death education will benefit them at their stage of life. Many palliative care services may not have the resources to service this particular population, but it is worth making the theoretical point that health promoting palliative care is not care that is necessarily, by definition, confined only to those with a terminal or obviously life-threatening illness.

Health promotion is a regular set of services provided by community health centres. The incorporation of death-awareness and education programs can easily help partly to convert conventional health promotion programs into health promoting palliative care services for older people. This is something that local palliative care services might encourage in their professional relationships with those services.

Aside from 'mainstreaming' health promoting palliative care principles through community health outlets, palliative care services might still legitimately ask who should be eligible for their particular offerings. In the first instance, health promoting palliative care programs are most suitable for people who, in the early stages of their disease, are currently well and ambulant. Clearly, some of the health education activities that require people to travel for second opinions, to seek complementary therapies, or to visit the offices of lawyers or accountants are best undertaken by people who already enjoy a reasonable level of fitness and health.

The above comments notwithstanding, much education and information about one's health can be gained by sitting in front of a computer screen and 'surfing' the Internet. There are a great many websites providing health information and networks, not to mention 'chat' sites to swap information or experiences. And even those who are computer illiterate, or bed-ridden, or both, are not excluded from any of these sources of education and information, because it is always possible to provide such information verbally on a one-to-one basis.

While most palliative care practitioners may have no trouble at all in supplying or facilitating health information for clients, some people may have concerns about providing death education. What, for example, if the person living with a terminal illness displays a reluctance to discuss topics related to death and dying? The idea that many individuals deny death is, at best, an unhelpful one. At worst, the idea of denial can be stigmatising and belittling. Instead, one should keep in mind the simpler idea that many people do not wish to talk about all things with all people. Instead, they *select* who is 'right' for particular kinds of confidences and discussions. If some people do not wish to discuss death with you, do not assume that they will not talk to others. If you suspect that this might be the situation, then perhaps you could refer the person to others for this discussion, or deal with the topic in group situations instead.

We must also remember the issue of timing. Some days are better than others for raising some topics. On some days, talk of death is depressing. At other times, a person may have a pressing need to talk about death, or dying, or both. The task of someone providing health promoting palliative care is to be ready and to appear, as best as they are able, responsive and informed about this topic.

At what stage of an illness?

Health promoting palliative care in the form of education and information, supports, and interpersonal reorientation should be supplied across the course of an illness. Naturally, the social, psychological, and spiritual issues will arise immediately after diagnosis—or sometimes, in the case of metastatic cancer, after the first reoccurrence—but the sooner these are addressed the better.

One of the most important reasons for supplying information and encouraging people to be active in their own self-education about health and medical matters is to create and enhance a genuine basis for 'informed' consent when people are confronted with treatment decisions. But the other rationale for providing this kind of support throughout the illness is the need to cultivate and actively support the experience of *hope* in all people with a life-threatening or terminal illness. In the context of serious illness, there are at least four kinds of hope. These can be found individually, or combined, across the course of all life-threatening or terminal illnesses.

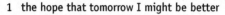

1 the hope that tomorrow I might be better
2 the hope that I might find daily or weekly satisfactions
3 the hope that I might leave something of lasting value to others
4 the hope that I might survive or transcend the present suffering

It is in the pursuit of these hopes that the direct service functions of health promoting palliative care become meaningful for many of the participants. Since these hopes arise during the entire course of a life-threatening or terminal illness, the implementation of these services should similarly follow the course of that illness.

People's hope that they might be better in fact, or at least feel better, or even look better for others, is one important motivation for embracing health promotion. An easing of symptoms, or perhaps the pursuit of remission, or the desire to stay in remission, is a laudable aim for health promotion that uses medical interventions or complementary therapies. Health maintenance is also a way of achieving daily satisfactions, such as being able to walk a certain distance unassisted, or to live long enough to be there for a nephew's birthday, or to keep that glass of red wine down long enough to savour it. Health helps one achieve a wide variety of goals associated with personal or social satisfaction. Health promoting palliative care is designed to enhance these.

An important social value of death education is its ability to help people to come to terms with 'life' after death. I mean this in two ways.

First, many people have a strong desire to leave something behind that will be of value to others. Sometimes this is simply a legal will that allocates personal effects to family and friends. At other times, people may wish to be of value by bequeathing their bodies to 'science'. Or at other times, they may participate in experimental therapies to help others. I knew a woman whose idea of leaving something of herself behind was knitting and crafting dolls (seventy in all) to give to as many people as she could. Finding the way and wherewithal to be a part of the lives of others after death is an important function of death education for people at any stage of their illness.

The second sense of 'life' after death is its usual meaning: the idea of personal survival beyond biological death itself. I realise that this is a sensitive and controversial issue nowadays. However, the reality is that most people have a belief in this kind of life after death. No doubt, some will celebrate, perhaps glibly, their appointment with extinction and oblivion. Very many more will wish to talk to clergy for an update on salvation. Still others will want to read an account of the debate over near-death experiences. A health promoting palliative care is about supplying information, or sources of information, that might aid in a person's own individual quest for understanding. The intellectual 'party lines' on these matters are irrelevant to most people.

In what manner?

The ideal professional style of health promoting palliative care should be participatory and discursive. In other words, one should aim for a balance between times devoted to organised and predetermined opportunities for learning and obtaining information, *and* other times devoted to exploring client-driven concerns. The reason for this balance is simple enough: not every person is aware of what he or she wants or needs to know.

Initially, it will be important to discover the range of needs that particular clients bring to the service; they may wish to know about the range of complementary therapies in their town; they may wish to join a support group; they may want to receive some information about their illness or about treatment programs. But after addressing their immediate or presenting needs, you will need to explain the full range of health promoting services that you offer.

Some of the education and information functions might take the form of monthly lectures in health or death education, particularly if the health promoting palliative care program is offered by an institution such as a hospital, hospice, or community health centre. Clients might develop other interests or needs based on what they learn in these more formal learning situations. Even here, though, 'lectures' should be brief, with *at least half* the allocated time being set aside for discussion of the material.

If the health promoting palliative care is being offered by an individual—such as by the local minister, for example—the principle remains much the same. An overview of what that practitioner is offering should occur initially. There will be times of discussion and other times when an overview, either of services or information, will need to be provided, followed by discussion opportunities related to that information. Nevertheless, a 'feedback loop' should always be maintained. The practitioner first listens to the initial needs, addresses those needs and provides new information, assesses any new needs and addresses those, and so on. Needs assessment should be ongoing, not only as part of any program evaluation, but also as a way of continually adhering to the ideal of client-driven programming.

Apart from listening to client *needs*, the other important insight to gain from listening to clients is to identify the shape, format, and content of health and death education opportunities themselves. Clearly, not all cancer diseases generate the same issues for all people. Cancer and cancer treatments are different from HIV and the treatment regimes for that disease. The health promoting issues for people with HIV may be different from those for clients with motor neurone disease.

Furthermore, younger people may seek different kinds of information in relation to death and dying than that sought by older people.

And despite the fact that social, psychological, and spiritual issues remain as urgent or as pressing as always across the course of a disease, degrees of physical disablement can fluctuate, creating different problems at different times. In the context of this diversity, the term 'needs' should be interpreted broadly, with some of this insight coming from clients themselves but other information being derived from social and physical observation.

PROVIDING SOCIAL SUPPORTS—PERSONAL AND COMMUNITY

The provision of social supports should be a process of strengthening existing relationships and developing new ones that are able to enhance a sense of well-being. These are steps that are crucial to the creation of health promoting environments at the close personal level. Personal supports can be strengthened by providing opportunities to meet others in the same situation, as well as by enlisting the support of friends and family.

Social supports should emerge from:
- people in a similar situation
- family and friends
- the wider community

People in similar situations

Learning takes place not only in formal talks or through reading and listening to informational material; support groups are also good places for clients to learn about their new situation and to team up with other members to solve problems or address issues of concern to them. Wherever possible, or whenever relevant, support groups should be encouraged to be self-care groups, helping members to address the needs that arise from their group meetings.

Support groups, therefore, may serve several functions. They may provide sources of genuine empathy and understanding from others who are in the same situation. Members can provide motivation and encouragement for each other. Such groups can provide a forum for joint problem-solving by bringing together people who are experienced in the problems themselves. They can provide group resources for the organisation and attainment of solutions. They provide a wider pool of people to share information and among whom to divide the labour for set tasks.

Family and friends

As with all palliative care services, family and friends can be involved if the client so wishes. There are several obvious ways that friends and family may participate in health promoting palliative care.

First, they can attend the support groups themselves. However, you may need to consider how often family and friends are able to attend these groups. Remember also that some people with life-threatening or terminal illnesses encounter problems with the very friends and family 'who dearly want to help'. Opportunities for the client to speak freely *without* the presence of family or their usual friends could also be important. Furthermore, for many clients, just saying that they do not want friends or family to be involved can itself be a problem, both socially (in giving offence) and personally (in feeling guilt for thinking or giving expression to these thoughts). It might be wise to develop a policy that certain sessions are for clients only—for example, every second or third session. On the other hand, family and friends themselves may need their own support. They might also appreciate opportunities of talking to people in the same circumstances as themselves. They might benefit from their own structured opportunities to talk—from their own support groups.

A second way that family and friends might become involved, aside from group work, is with the gathering of information for the client.

Family and friends whose idea of 'helping' is 'doing something' might be encouraged to help with information seeking and gathering. They might use their personal computers to trawl the Internet for information on behalf of their friend, or even their friend's support group. They can act as research assistants too, collecting brochures from lawyers, funeral directors, or meditation services for the perusal of the client and his or her support group.

Third, friends and family can participate in the death education program, whatever shape this takes. As I argued earlier, death education is for anyone facing death, and by definition, that is all of us. There is no reason why discussion of death—either the social preparations for death or the religious issues—should not be of value to everyone. Resuscitation and first aid are not only taught to those who might have obvious need to use them. They are promoted to everyone, because anyone may need these skills at some time or another. So it is with death education.

Finally, friends and family can be involved, at home or at work, with any of the lifestyle changes that the client needs to make. In this regard, family and friends can help with dietary changes or changes in lifestyle to accommodate exercise (or extra exercise) the introduction of meditation regimes, or visits to complementary therapists. In addition to these voluntary changes, family, friends, and especially work mates might need to make allowances for the client, whose bouts of tiredness or weakness may require time out during the day or a change in work tasks.

Community

The general community can also contribute and should be encouraged to contribute to health promoting care in its capacity to support the person with a life-threatening or terminal illness. Support groups are only one type of support for clients, and a limited one at that. There are several ways the general community can provide important support.

First, community groups can help with funding. A library, the cost of audio tapes, and even sessional staff all require some kind of ongoing budget. Core costs may be supported by an institution's palliative care budget, but it is just as likely that this will not be the case, or that extra funds are needed in order to extend the service to become a health promoting one. Business groups, service associations such as Rotary or Apex, and local church or school organisations can help with sponsorship, donations, or fund-raising.

Second, local groups can also help supply information and education sources, depending on the need. In my city, for example, a funeral business has one of the largest and best stocked libraries of books on the subject of death and dying. My own university holds all the main academic and professional journals on death, dying, and grief. Arrangements can be made for general members of the community to borrow from these libraries. There are also specialist New Age book stores, which might supply catalogues for those who have an interest in that area.

Municipal libraries might be asked to contribute a list of relevant holdings that relate to diseases and their treatments, death, dying and bereavement, health promotion, or books related to getting one's 'affairs in order'. There may also be useful video material in the form of documentaries on euthanasia, near-death experiences, or world religions. Local libraries are also useful places to obtain interlibrary loans from other libraries all over the country.

There are a range of existing services for grief support or chronic illness support. Community health centres will have much of this information and should be encouraged to network with a health promoting service and to be active within it. Above and beyond their usual health and welfare services, local councils might also be invited to contribute in more imaginative but no less useful ways to support those with serious illnesses. They might, for example, think about the role of animal companions in the lives of people with serious illnesses. They could provide animals as temporary companions from their local pounds, or they could provide temporary relief support for people's own pets. They might also provide supportive suggestions about providing for people's pets when the owners are no longer able to care for them, particularly for people who live alone. Arrangements to transfer the pets to minders or new owners might help in some situations.

Community groups might also contribute speakers from a range of areas that might interest those living with a life-threatening or terminal illness. Local lawyers or accountants, for example, might be encouraged to give a little of their time to group sessions or small lectures on financial and legal issues relevant to death.

Media sources in the community might perform two important functions for health promoting palliative care. They may help publicise the health promoting service and its philosophy, thereby assisting the service with self-referrals. Second, popular media may also bring the social, personal, and spiritual issues pertinent to death and dying into sharper focus within the community. They may help raise these issues and thereby help reduce their 'dark' and marginal status, by blending them into everyday concerns. Media attention can contribute to the 'normalising' of human concern with death and dying, and to the community support and care of the dying.

ENCOURAGING INTERPERSONAL REORIENTATION

Through the use of support groups, and educational and informational opportunities, people with life-threatening or terminal illnesses might be encouraged to cope with changes and problems in their current situation.

Interpersonal reorientation can be encouraged through:
- support groups
- health education
- death education

- social information and education
- directory of services
- library resources

Support groups

I have already described how support groups might operate in terms of sharing experience, information, resources, and tasks. The primary purpose of such experiences is to encourage interpersonal reorientation. In these informal groups, members are able to swap experiences and share problems that relate to their illnesses. Other members—who may be more or less experienced—may make suggestions on how to solve these problems.

Some members may help others anticipate and/or prepare for social and personal situations that have not yet been encountered, such as friends or family members being over-protective, a sharp rise in social popularity, or stigma and rejection from work mates. Others may have 'good' accountants or solicitors who they can recommend; or they may have tried a certain practitioner of meditation or a naturopath who they highly regard and can recommend.

Groups can also provide a forum in which to discuss weekly or monthly reading or lecture material about health promotion, lifestyle change, or spiritual issues. An individual rarely has the time to read everything, and so different group members may read different kinds of books or arguments about the one topic and come together to share and debate the various issues. Changes in a person's spiritual orientation may be brought about by this kind of group work.

Education and information

In laying the foundations for personal change, the content of information and education programs is a crucial practice issue. There are several broad content areas that should be covered. These are, broadly:

- health information related to diet and exercise
- a critical appraisal of alternative ideas about healing terminal illnesses, such as vitamins and herbal remedies, meditation, faith healing, and many other ideas that are subject to medical suspicion
- the role of complementary therapy
- alternative medical approaches to certain life-threatening and terminal illnesses
- information about a person's illness and about treatment ideas

Another important form of health education will be to review sources of social information about living with chronic illness and dying. There are several useful books—both popular and academic—on living with HIV or cancer; there are also several equally revealing books on the medical, psychological, and social problems of the dying process, examining dying from prognosis to the final hours. If a group or individual feels that this information is important to their sense of preparedness, these references, or summaries of this information, might be kept in some accessible form.

Death education topics might include:

- a review of ideas about life after death for different religions
- a review of death-related research concerning personal survival of death (for example, near-death experiences, near-death visions, visions of the bereaved, and so on)
- social preparations for death, including information and educational sessions on legal and financial preparations
- funeral preparations
- interpersonal preparations
- donations of organs to others (usually not appropriate) or to medical institutions
- ideas about social or material forms of legacy

These, and other possible topics, can be covered in a variety of ways. Obviously, some of this material can be covered in lectures or seminars.

It might also be covered by using reading lists. Some of the information can be placed on audio or video tapes for borrowing. Local experts on different topics might be persuaded to talk on these tapes. A directory of services might also provide some of this material. A critical guide to 'alternative' or complementary services might contain a list of all such practitioners in town, with a description of what they offer and critical remarks about price, safety, and past client opinions. A similar guide could be compiled for other services, such as funeral or legal services. If possible, a library could be set up in the hospice, or the existing library could be expanded to include health promoting or death-related material. Lone practitioners could perhaps make an arrangement with the local library, whereby a special health education or death education bibliography is compiled for the use of health promoting palliative care users.

REORIENTATION OF PALLIATIVE CARE SERVICES

Aside from providing support groups, the reorientation of health services is also integral to the creation of supportive environments in the wider sense. There are three key ways in which one might encourage a reorientation of palliative care services towards a health promoting philosophy and service. These approaches include professional development and education, research, and policy development.

Reorient palliative care services through:
- tertiary education and training
- links to public-health associations and professionals
- research into the early stages of dying
- policy analysis

The initial and most basic form of professional education and development occurs during the tertiary training of students. Where 'palliative care' is taught at an undergraduate level, the core principles of a health promoting palliative care should be introduced. If 'palliative care' is not offered at undergraduate level (and, in the 'helping professions', it is difficult to imagine why it would not be, at least as an elective offering), then some introduction to the issues surrounding 'death, dying, and grief' or similar subject should be given, and should include some health promoting ideas.

The subject of 'death and dying' should not be treated in undergraduate courses only in terms of 'loss'—an idea from studies of grief and bereavement that seems to have spread, without critical checks, to the topic of dying. Dying is only sometimes about loss and just as much about other experiences, including health. This idea should be strongly emphasised and linked to subjects such as 'death and dying' so that students might see dying as part of living.

At graduate or postgraduate levels, all palliative care subjects should include the core principles of health promoting palliative care. Social work courses might also explore how a model of health promoting palliative care might fit with the prevailing models of social case-work, group work, and community work. Pastoral care courses might do the same, but in relation to churches' own models of counselling and parish work.

In addition to the standard postgraduate courses that are offered in order to meet different occupational requirements in relation to palliative care, each of these areas might be encouraged to view postgraduate degrees in public health as relevant qualifications in palliative care. On its own, a specialisation in health promotion can be a valuable qualification for workers who wish to develop health promoting palliative care programs. It may also be an extremely relevant additional qualification for those who already hold standard graduate qualifications in palliative care within their own professional areas (for example, in medicine or nursing).

Professionals already practising palliative care might also consider joining the local public health or health promotion association in their state or county, using these associations' journals and professional meetings as useful sources of professional development in palliative care.

Research is another important and crucial way of reorienting palliative care services. This research should continue the tradition of health services research that is already evident in the palliative care literature, but should also extend into the areas of dying, and living with dying. Most of the literature in current palliative care journals is about the dying, but the voice of the dying is difficult to discern. There are 'needs' surveys and there are 'case studies', but there is little work examining the social life of people living with terminal or life-threatening illness.

Furthermore, much of the research about dying is problem-based, focusing on areas that may be troublesome for the dying and for their carers. But life, and living with dying, involves more than just troubles. It is important to identify issues that are important to living with dying, and to understand how an illness, such as HIV or cancer, can shape one's experience with carers and one's usual life concerns. Without this attention to the 'normal', we will constantly portray serious illness simply and tragically as a 'problem time'—something for the community, and professionals, genuinely to fear and dread.

The above comments notwithstanding, there is still much need to research the social and psychological issues relating to the *early* part of dying—from prognosis to disablement. Once again, our attention has focused on the stage of the serious illness that gives clinicians most concern. This is an unbalanced research agenda. Furthermore, the picture of serious illness remains heavily slanted towards issues of biology and illness instead of more positively towards social experiences and personal identity. Research in the latter areas is needed to restore a balance to our understanding of dying. Only when these issues are given significant priority in the research agendas of palliative care will palliative care services be reoriented towards health promotion.

Finally, policy development that might expand the reach of palliative care services, and the extra funding needed for such an expansion, can only come about if it is supported and linked to research. Practice and policy must be evidence-based because, aside from the politics of policy development, it is research evidence that impresses both communities and funding bodies. Support for any policy to reorient palliative care towards health promotion will be based on evidence that demonstrates the need for these developments.

Furthermore, there are currently policy gaps that might be demonstrated to municipal, state, and national government departments. Conventional palliative care services in most countries are very much geared towards serious and disabling illness and not towards early periods of wellness. Given the openness of palliative care services to servicing this period, and to accepting the principles of health promotion, what reasons might governments have for refusing to increase funding for early-stage palliative care services? Existing policies should be examined in the light of this question.

Clearly, there will be funding pressures. Nevertheless, policy issues regarding priority areas within palliative care and/or public health itself may require review and research. Accepting that palliative care has a public health mission and agenda entails a claim on public health resources and the policy developments relevant to this mission. Only palliative care practitioners and researchers can pursue this policy development. The reorientation of these practitioners is vital if policy developments in the broader public health arena are to follow.

COMBATING DEATH-DENYING HEALTH POLICIES AND ATTITUDES

In general, it is not true or helpful to say that we live in a 'death-denying' society. We do not. Death and dying are recognised. The book you are reading is evidence enough of that. Businesses and professions are organised around these events and experiences. Some small interest groups in society, the cryogenics society for example, may be death-denying, but their presence in no way makes the wider society death-denying.

Nevertheless, most people's waking lives are not given much to thinking about death or dying unless they are directly affected by these experiences. In the main, people and their activities are life-affirming. Few would argue that it should be otherwise. However, the absence of thinking about death and dying on the part of most people does itself mean that people are usually poorly prepared for death and dying, be it their own or other people's. This is the wider context of death-denying social attitudes and practices. People 'deny' only in the sense of rarely thinking about or acting on the idea of death. Since health professionals are people, most professionals not working in palliative care are part of this problem of apathy with regard to death.

The first strategy to combat this problem, then, is to reorient conventional health services towards the idea of death and dying. Part of how this might be achieved has already been covered in my comments about research and tertiary training. In the wider community, however, more direct approaches might be considered. Health promoting palliative care services might provide death education nights or seminars for the general public. These could be free, or low-cost, and could be conducted quarterly as a general community-education service. Such seminars are also a useful way to encourage community interest in the palliative care service, a source of community recruitment of volunteers, and valuable networks for identifying lesser known informational, educational, and funding resources. I have already commented on the usefulness of regular relationships with the media—print, television, and radio. These organisations have powerful access to the community's ears and eyes, and are invaluable generators of self-referrals for the palliative care service itself.

In addition to tertiary training for professionals (degree and diploma courses), the community will directly benefit from short courses and adult-education courses conducted by local adult- and community-education institutions. Some of these will be supported and run by local technical and further education institutions, but could also be run by adult-education bodies, or in high schools that hire their premises to worthy educational agencies.

Community involvement is also crucial in breaking down death-denying attitudes. In this respect, volunteers might play an important role as research assistants to self-help or support groups. Volunteers can be of enormous assistance in gathering information, arranging speakers, or simply transporting valuable educational items (audio tapes, books, and so on) to groups.

Health professionals should also be encouraged to participate in health promoting services. In public health areas, professionals might explore staff exchanges on a fractional, part-time, or sessional basis. This might also help with issues of staff 'burn-out' within the areas of both palliative care and public health. In any case, as mentioned earlier, community health centres might be valuable sources of collaboration for palliative care practitioners once the principles of health promoting palliative care have been discussed by the two service areas.

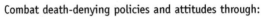

Combat death-denying policies and attitudes through:
- lay seminars
- media relationships
- short courses
- community involvement (for example, volunteers)
- staff exchanges

OTHER DEVELOPMENT ISSUES—THE FURTHER IMPORTANCE OF RESEARCH

Aside from the practice principles involved in meeting the main goals of a health promoting palliative care, there are other issues related to the development of such programs that require brief discussion. These include:

- variations on the model
- the rationale behind the broad development of all core concerns
- the applicability of conventional health promotion problems to a health promoting palliative care

These concerns centre in great part around the priority accorded to research in health promoting palliative care.

Variations on the model

The core concerns of health promoting palliative care are health education, death education, social supports, interpersonal reorientation, and environmental and policy development. Although these program offerings are delivered in concert with each other, the emphasis on individual components will vary somewhat from program to program.

Clearly, any variations on the model of health promoting palliative care will depend mostly on whether this type of care is offered by an individual (by a private practitioner or chaplain) or an institution (for example, a hospice). The major issues underlying the core concerns of the model are education, support, and research and policy development. While there are numerous ways to facilitate support as a lone practitioner or an institution, difficulties might occur in relation to educational and research facilities and capacities.

The health promoting palliative care offered by hospitals or hospices might be expected to have some advantages over lone practitioner services in terms of infrastructure. For example, institutions are more likely to have lecture or seminar rooms available for larger group functions. Apart from being able to provide space for support groups to meet, these areas might also be large enough for lectures or meetings for community groups. Lecture rooms, apart from being suitable for health and death education lecture opportunities, might also be useful for adult-education sessions, fund-raising meetings, or small conference meetings. An institution is also more likely to have its own library, which might be adapted for client use by expanding the collection, or extending the borrowing privileges, or both.

Institutions are also places where it is likely that more than one staff member will have an interest in palliative care and, therefore, where research groups are more likely to develop. This is extremely important to the policy-development aspects of the model. Furthermore, once a group of researchers is established, networks with other researchers in the same city or state can be developed more efficiently. It is more likely that at least one person from the group will always be able to attend seminars at neighbouring universities or be able to meet with others to swap information, attend short courses, or establish collaborations with relevant expertise.

If you are providing health promoting palliative care as a lone practitioner, some of these achievements are not as easy to accomplish. It might be a good idea to think about how information is to be supplied to clients. Lectures for audiences of less than ten or twenty people can be awkward. You might want to think about a reading list that you can use to guide people through the issues, and as a basis for subsequent meetings and discussion. For those people who do not find reading appealing, you might consider creating a set of audio tapes to which clients and their families can listen.

If you do not have a library, you might consider linking up with local municipal, hospital, or university libraries to support your services. Policy- or practice-relevant research may not be easy to conduct alone. If research and writing do not come easily to you, collaboration may be the answer. You might approach local palliative care services and invite those interested in health promoting palliative care to attend a 'research meeting' that you organise at your premises. Here, you might meet regularly to discuss the policy and practice issues relevant to all group members. Team research might emerge from these talks, and a division of labour that addresses and uses each person's particular strengths and training may emerge.

Why development of *all* core concerns

Clearly, education and support groups are the strategies with which most health professionals will be most comfortable. The goals of these strategies are readily identified and understood. Most professionals are equipped with the relevant training and experience. But research and policy development are areas in which perhaps not everyone will be equally at ease. Nevertheless, the development of these areas is particularly important to health promotion in general, and health promoting palliative care in particular. There are six reasons for believing this to be so.

First, research is about learning new things and communicating those findings. It is a social act that is aimed at self and community improvement. When clients come to access information on the topics of health or death, they are engaging in a form of research. In order to provide the best, most up-to-date facts, opinions, or arguments for these clients, it is incumbent upon staff to engage in the same process.

Second, policy development is partly determined by networks, but also by access to facts, new insights, or arguments. The research act itself is a most powerful and persuasive tool for policy development. The act of establishing a 'need' for some new service, facility, or funding is best achieved by providing 'evidence' of that 'need'. Research can supply that evidence.

Third, all personal experience is limited. Research can force our professional gaze to be systematic and thorough. It can put professional 'reins' on professional 'impressions' by encouraging us to check the numbers, to observe more closely, or to dwell or think more deeply about a particular experience. In other words, research can improve professional practice.

Fourth, we are long past the time when our own positive impressions were enough to justify to anyone that we were offering a service that was relevant to our governments, communities, profession, or clients. An evaluation strategy that monitors the quality and relevance of our services is now essential for both credibility and quality assurance. Evaluation, if properly performed, is a form of research.

Fifth, if we believe that health promoting palliative care is an important model of palliative care, then the onus will be on us to demonstrate the value of such programs, their ability to address the social character of living with dying, and their active, participatory, and health promoting effectiveness. Published research is one of the most enduring means of establishing these goals.

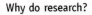

Why do research?
- responsibilities to clients
- policy development
- improves professional knowledge and practice
- quality assurance
- demonstrates to others the value of health promoting palliative care
- monitors problems / solves problems

Health promotion problems revisited

The final reason why the research functions of a health promoting palliative care are crucial is that they enable practitioners to monitor and avoid the problems that have occasionally arisen in other health promotion programs. The most obvious problem is that environmental and policy initiatives have often taken second place. If health is part of the wider network of concerns in a person's life—including work, religion, family, and sexual relationships—then policy initiatives to enhance health must be accompanied by research and initiatives in those areas.

If we are to avoid naive interpersonal interventions that inadvertently discriminate against others or reinforce or reproduce inequalities in other parts of society, then we must use penetrating, critical tools that can steer us away from these mistakes. Good research can provide us with that quality assurance.

Overall, the key means to achieve the goals of health promoting palliative care are to design and adopt services that provide health and death education, social supports, interpersonal reorientation, and environmental and policy development. Exactly how we might go about designing these offerings, and the rationale for doing so, are subjects for the remaining chapters. The next chapter will begin by examining the issues relevant to health education.

3

Health Education

By health I mean

the power to live a full, adult, living, breathing life

in close contact with what I love

Katherine Mansfield, as quoted in

Murry 1983, p. 254

This chapter represents the first of two chapters dedicated to a discussion and introduction of educational programming in health promoting palliative care. Health and death education are health promoting activities that are governed by similar philosophies and strategies. In death education, it is relatively easy to outline relevant content areas since the broad concerns about death and dying are similar for everyone. For health education, however, it is not possible to be prescriptive about content areas for obvious reasons. People who enter palliative care present with a diverse array of diseases, and each of these entail different illness experiences, therapies, and side-effects. In this chapter, therefore, I will describe the major strategies for educational programs, remembering that these strategies apply to both health and death education programs. Each of these strategies can be applied or employed with information and knowledge about different diseases when this information is at hand.

I organise the chapter in the following way. First, I will broadly examine the rival theories of health education as they exist in the current literature. I will spend a brief time reflecting on the dilemma we face when attempting to choose between them, and then I will offer a way forward. Second, I will outline and discuss the process issues involved in the delivery of any health promoting education program, bearing in mind that the basic assumption underlying such programs is the need for a participatory approach. Finally, I will summarise the major and most popular strategies used in health education programs the world over.

THEORIES, THEORIES, THEORIES . . .

As soon as we turn our attention to the problem of changing people's behaviour, we immediately encounter the theories of psychology. This is particularly obvious when we discuss therapy of any kind, and this is because we need to ask (and get an answer to) the question 'What types of experiences, events or influences will help people to change?'

Because health education has been primarily concerned with motivating people to achieve good health, much of its efforts have been focused on getting people to change. Theories about the self, then, have preoccupied some health educators. Helen Ross and Paul Mico (1980), for example, have summarised some of the theories that might be relevant to health education because most health education strategies assume that people are 'built' in a certain way.

Personality theory assumes that people are reflective and rational— that they are capable of making choices. Developmental theory adds the idea that people may indeed be rational and reflective but that different issues are important to different people at different ages. Motivational theories argue that the ruling influence in people's lives is not necessarily age, but rather it is the satisfaction of basic needs. People are only motivated to spend considerable time philosophising, for example, if their food and shelter requirements are satisfied first. Learning theory argues that, age and motivation notwithstanding, people can learn most things if the conditions are conducive enough. Group theories add that, since so much learning takes place in groups, groups themselves are crucial for personal change. And, of course, psychoanalytic theories argue that past relationships and learning can be highly influential on present and future ones. Moreover, people are not necessarily rational. People can be clearly, or not so clearly, defensive.

But in the final analysis, each of these theories offers the health educator basic parameters for thinking about certain groups and fields. Each individual, and each group, has its own reasons for acting, believing, and thinking in the way that it does. Health educators employ theories of self as prompts or guides to thinking about the individual or group before them. Listening, reflecting, and checking back with the individual or group about what motivates them and what does not is the only reliable guide. This observation seems a simple one to make, but it is often ignored when we move to theories of health education. Here, the stakes seem higher.

There are three major models of health education. The first model is the individualist model of health education, also known as the 'health-ism model', the 'conservative model', the 'medical model', or the 'pre-ventative model'. (For a review of these models, see French & Adams 1986; Tones et al. 1990; and Colquhoun 1991.) In the individualist model, the emphasis is on changing the individual's behaviour. The individual should give up smoking, fatty foods, a sedentary lifestyle, work stress; he or she should take up exercise, eat more vegetables, and practise relaxation. The emphasis is on changing the attitudes and behaviours of people who sit before the health educators' very eyes. It has been criticised for being 'victim-blaming'—that is, for placing the responsibility for illness on individuals instead of the social and political system of the day. Better driving techniques, for example, do not over-come the effects of poor roads or poorly built motor vehicles.

The radical–political model, also known as the 'structuralist model', takes the opposite view of health education, arguing that useful health education is consciousness-raising, encouraging people to look at the social and political conditions that shape their health and illness in everyday life. Health education, then, should be based on community action and not simply about 'changing attitudes'. Derek Colquhoun (1991) argues that this is a paternalistic approach and deprives ordinary individuals of any sense of agency and control. It is true that structural models do not blame the individual. Rather, the individual is rendered invisible in the analysis.

Finally, Keith Tones, Sylvia Tilford, and Yvonne Robinson (1990) describe the self-empowerment model. Rather than assuming that people need to be told what to do by radical community workers or conservative health professionals, the idea behind this model is to max-imise participant choice. Participants are encouraged to clarify their personal beliefs and values. They are also encouraged to recognise barriers to their choices (for example, class, upbringing, drugs of addiction, and so on), and this model aims to assist them directly in overcoming these barriers in whatever way is relevant to them. This might involve community action. It might involve individual counselling. It is the participants, however, who are the final arbiters of their needs, rather than the particular *a priori* beliefs of the practitioner.

I have taken the trouble to briefly summarise these theories of self- and health education because I assume that most readers will see the wisdom of making client needs and characteristics the central guide in selecting their practice style. Many people who work in nursing, medicine, or social work might readily see in the two extreme health education examples that the only way to avoid the paternalism of both approaches is to check and re-check *one's own bias and preferences* about health care. This conclusion may not seem surprising, but it seems that it is easier to make in academic contexts than in practical ones. Let us look at cancer care as an example of what I mean here.

In the care of people who are seriously ill with cancer, we can identify at least three enthusiastic and protective (perhaps paternalistic) views: the medical perspective, the New Age perspective, and the critical public health perspective.

The medical perspective naturally strongly endorses its own therapies: chemotherapy, radiotherapy, surgery, and so on. Its assumptions and confidence derive from faith in an empirically based, positivist tradition of science. The medical view is that you can believe what you like about stress, the influence of the mind, or Laetrile, but a randomised control trial (RCT), the 'gold standard' of medical research methodology, should and will be the final arbiter. Medical therapy may not have the answers, but you can be sure that the complementary people do not have them yet either.

However, with some notable exceptions, little harm can come from complementary therapies, and some improvement in the quality of living with cancer might be gained. It is not recommended that people with life-threatening illnesses avoid conventional medical treatment, whatever complementary advice they receive. Many so-called 'recoveries' or 'cures' often turn out to be premature declarations, were the result of earlier conventional treatments or wrong diagnoses, or are a one-in-100 000 case of spontaneous remission (Buckman 1996).

On the other hand, New Age perspectives regard complementary therapy highly. We do not know everything there is to know, or we would have a cure for cancer. Medicine, too, is not omniscient. Medicine has not made major inroads into the mortality or morbidity rates of most of the major cancers, despite the multi-billion-dollar industry of research that supports it.

As for rigorous research designs such as the RCT, any methodologist can identify a series of problems with these that is as long as your weekly shopping list. Many RCTs are too complex, inconclusive, or unethical to be taken seriously, leading some to argue that the RCT, as a reliable, revealing method, is 'dead' (Herman 1995). More specifically, others have argued that, while participants in RCTs are randomised, their selection for inclusion into the study itself is usually not random. This is called 'sample bias' and is a recognised problem of this research design. It is a particular problem in cancer treatments, where research into participant characteristics (see Gotay 1991) has shown that non-participation is strongly influenced by physician and patient characteristics. Generalisations from these studies are highly dubious and restricted (see Daly et al. 1997).

On the other hand, there are a good many published accounts of people who have broken away from conventional medical treatments and who have succeeded in curing themselves. Is it just the luck of one in 100 000? Maybe it is, but so few people have the courage and support in such desperate times to free themselves from medical ideas that this figure may simply represent the low-tide mark of those willing to try. Perhaps.

The critical public-health perspective argues that both the above perspectives are missing the point. The search for a 'magic bullet' is an example of 'down-stream' thinking. Healers, both medical and complementary, are pulling drowning people out of the river as fast as they can. But the 'real' problem is up-stream. Who, or what, is throwing them into the river in the first place?

This analogy also applies to biological explanations. The discovery of organic hypotheses for cancer aetiology does not minimise the importance of environmental factors, and these factors—smoking in the workplace, the widespread use of alcohol as a stress-reducing, relaxation practice, and so on—are social and political issues. These are the issues that should be given priority in health action and spending. When a person with carcinoma of the lung appears in the waiting room of a general practitioner, the major damage has already been done. We are now in 'last resort' territory—secondary or tertiary intervention, complementary or medical. Serious health care is political health care.

Each of these three perspectives has strong evidence and even stronger arguments to support it. You might recognise your particular bias by your attraction to one of the individual summaries above. The fact is that most seriously ill people do not have time to argue or work out for themselves whether the 'medicalisation of everyday life' arguments of the New Age or critical public-health people have merit, or whether 'doctor still knows best'. Time is running out—fast.

We are all located at the very centre of our own reading and experiences—all convinced of the rightness and worth of our considered opinions. In health care, we are all keen to protect and support our clients to the best of that knowledge and experience. Like parents who love their adult children, we can regularly forget that they are not children at all, but adults. This is what is meant by paternalism.

How do we move beyond these three perspectives without abandoning the value and worth of their insights? There is no doubt at all that health has a political side to its aetiology, and health promoting palliative care recognises this dimension in its environmental and policy approach (see chapter 7). There is a place for institutional and community strategies, and these occupy a privileged place in health promotion in general. In this chapter, however, we are focusing on one-on-one experiences of learning. This is not a conservative response but a practical 'housekeeping' one.

When we recognise that many of our health care practitioners are actually case workers, we simultaneously recognise that it is appropriate to spend significant time on strategies relevant to that form of care. This brings us to the observation made by Tones, Tilford, and Robinson (1990, p. 14) that when it comes to theoretical differences in outlook, 'quite substantial ideological differences may be reconciled in practice!' In other words, few people are active, competitive ideologues in practice, and different types of practitioners are frequently open to the possibilities offered by each other.

Nevertheless, the one commonality that characterises individual and institutional health care relationships, complementary or medical, is the traditional sick role. Patients and healers collaborate in an often taken-for-granted role play, in which patients 'need' and healers 'do'. Healers are 'consulted' and patients 'comply'. Healers are 'experts' and patients come for a 'prescription'. In other words, the barriers to acknowledging other ways of doing things are rarely in the knowledge, attitudes, or beliefs of practitioners, but rather they are part of the interpersonal processes of their practice. There is often much listening, and very much more advising, but less than ideal amounts of *facilitating*. And yet it is the process of facilitating the desires of people that most gives them a sense of hope, support, and control.

In health promoting palliative care, a care based on the principle of participatory social relations, we need to situate and recognise our biases, own up to them, and actively facilitate and encourage others to discover and pursue their own vision of health and meaning. This is the basic meaning of the goal of empowerment, and its most important message is this: the best health education is not simply to be found in the 'strategies' themselves but rather in the *processes* by which health education is learnt by those who come to it.

PROCESSES

Over the years, the World Health Organization (1988), UNICEF (n.d.), and health educationalists (Smyth 1986; Colquhoun 1991) have made a number of suggestions about how to implement a participatory style in health education programs. There are a good number of books that you might consult about this style of education. Nevertheless, we can identify some simple suggestions from the above authors and agencies that capture the spirit of how one should proceed.

The first and most obvious step to a participatory style is to listen to others. Listen carefully to people's presenting problems and the initial desires and hopes that they bring to you. Listening is quite a skill. Most people have an exaggerated view of their listening abilities. Listening is always assumed to be easy. I am constantly surprised by people I meet who can remember what particular points they disagree with in something they have read or heard, but who struggle to summarise accurately anything else from the same text or program. You can check if this applies to you by offering a brief summary of what you understand someone to have been saying ('paraphrasing') and checking how often you are accurate from that person's point of view.

Second, both you and the person with whom you are speaking should try to think about how any problems identified have been caused, might be cured, or might be prevented in the future. This might be simple. Problems might have been caused by a poor understanding of the disease. They might be the result of lack of clarity about treatment options.

Third, you might make an assessment of the person's current behaviour or problems that summarises the presenting situation for your own records. Here you need to learn about the person's current knowledge, beliefs, or behaviour as a starting point upon which you can build together, but also as a benchmark for future evaluation. Remember that evaluation is also part of your ongoing commitment in health promoting palliative care. You need to document the person's current problems and limitations in order to later assess how these have improved, or not, after contact with your program. At this point, you also need to investigate sources of information about the presenting health problem that may be of use to you both. You might here develop your new (and/or test your existing) educational materials and strategies. Each new person or group who uses these aids might challenge you to revise or modify them.

Next you might help people identify the reasons for their current actions and feelings. The educationalist John Smyth has some useful suggestions for how this might be achieved. As an example, you might ask, and explore the answers to, the following questions:

1 Where did the ideas I have about my illness/disease/future prospects come from historically?
2 How did I come to accept them?
3 Why do I continue to endorse them?
4 Whose interests are best served by them?
5 What power relations are involved?
6 How do these ideas shape and limit my current conduct?
7 In the light of my answers to the above questions, how may I now work/behave/feel differently?

Adapted from Smyth 1986

Medical writer Jeff Kane (1991, pp. 4–8; but see also Register 1989) begins from a similar starting point when he encourages his patients who have serious cancer to explore what he calls the '5 falsehoods':

1 You're a victim of cancer/stroke/HIV, and so on.
2 You'll be sick for the rest of your life.
3 There's no effective treatment for your illness.
4 You'll have a life expectancy of 6–12 months.
5 Your condition is terminal.

Other topics might also be included depending on what ideas are of particular concern to the people to whom you are listening. Sometimes this might be about treatment decisions, about how others believe someone with cancer or HIV should act, or about one's ambivalence about seeking a second medical opinion for fear of offending. The point to remember here is that a participatory health education is *reflective and critical*. For a participatory health education to be critical and reflective, it must encourage a rediscovery of the 'subject', the personal. In other words, practitioners need regularly to reflect on and seek to understand how their personal and professional backgrounds shape their responses, biases, and prejudices during the course of their care of people with serious illnesses.

Furthermore, participants should also be encouraged to seek actively to clarify their own personal needs and values and to pursue their own visions of 'health', 'quality of life', and/or 'control and empowerment'. It is not always clear *whose* ideas we hold, *why* we hold onto these ideas (particularly if and when they cease to serve us well), *how* these ideas limit or empower us, and *what* strategies we might employ to disentangle the threads of human socialisation. Nevertheless, if there is an attitude to be changed, it might be a person's attitude to received ideas, particularly those that appear to be oppressive.

After exploring the anatomy of received ideas, so to speak, the next step should be to encourage people to come up with their own ideas for solving the problem. Here, a group situation can be very useful. Groups can assist with 'brainstorming'—everyone pitching in with as many suggestions as possible, however wild or unusual. It is important to help people to look at their own ideas and to choose the most simple and most useful one(s) to put into practice. Clearly group meetings can be creative ways to generate suggestions, but patience, persistence, and spending time on a one-to-one basis can be as satisfactory. Always remember the culture from which the participant is from, and if people are to be enlisted for help, choose people who have credibility in the participant's eyes—not necessarily yours. In this way, you encourage people to use the ideas best suited to their backgrounds and circumstances.

STRATEGIES

We can speak of two kinds of strategies in health education. The first kind might be termed 'social strategies'. These are the strategies that you will find described in most health education or health promotion books: audiovisual aids, role plays, lectures, and so on. We need to review these because:

1 not everyone is familiar with the range of social strategies available to them to help others in their learning
2 these are important and basic technologies that have a long and useful history in education
3 these are the easiest and most commonly available media to employ for the purposes of health education—in palliative care or elsewhere

However, social strategies do not represent all the strategies that we might employ in health education. This is because a critical and reflective health education is one that takes the personal—the subjective experience of people—seriously. For the purposes of researching the self in relation to chronic and serious illness, there are a number of 'personal strategies'. The following two sections introduce some social and personal strategies that health promoting palliative care practitioners might find useful as a basic starting set of suggestions.

Social strategies

There are basically ten strategies that are relevant to working with individuals or groups for the purposes of health education. I draw these largely from the work of Mark Dignan and Patricia Carr (1987), Garry Egger, Ross Spark, and Jim Lawson (1990), and Jerrold Greenberg (1988). If you have experience with health education programs of any sort, you will be familiar with most of these strategies. What follows is a list and brief description of the main strategies, commenting on the space, evaluation, and labour implications of each.

Audiovisual aids

Examples of these aids include audio tapes, video tapes, books and articles, films, slides, posters, television, and of course, personal computers and their assorted software programs and compact disc options. As mentioned earlier, it is a good idea to establish a small library of health education material on the premises if at all possible. Participants can borrow materials from the library or skim the collection to decide if they wish to purchase or borrow another copy from elsewhere. An initial browse of your material might be important for potential clients of your service or practice. If you are unable to establish your own library, however modest, you might organise access to one in order to construct an annotated bibliography. Participants can use and think about this bibliography before visiting the library themselves. If borrowing rights are difficult to arrange, then at least you can direct participants to the library for on-site use.

Audiovisual materials have a particular advantage in complementing many other strategies; they can be used by those who enjoy reading or those who prefer to sit and watch information on television. The effectiveness of many of these kinds of strategies is also easy to evaluate. Depending on the size of a collection, there are obvious space requirements to be considered as well as costs to bear. These kinds of aids are also a little cerebral and can be asocial. However, if this material is used within a group context, audiovisual aids do not necessarily have these limitations. In general, the aids are easily used by institutions or by individual practitioners.

Counselling and behaviour modification

Sometimes people bring serious personal problems to their new situation. Following diagnosis, they may enter a deep depression, begin to have recurring anxiety attacks, or develop persistent anger with no apparent single target. Other people may suddenly have a strong desire to give up smoking or to overcome a long-term fear. Others encounter distressing problems in relation to their sexuality or to alcohol or drug use.

On these occasions, a health promoting palliative care may need to widen its resources and networks. If the program is run by an institution that has multi-professional staff, a therapist may be recommended to work with particular participants. If working as an individual practitioner, referral may be necessary. It is a good idea to keep a list of professionals whom you believe to be effective and experienced in relevant areas, particularly for people with serious illness. A participant might consult these people for advice or be fully referred to them if the participant considers this to be of value. Of course, counselling or therapy of any kind is labour-intensive for the staff involved, but its effectiveness is easy to evaluate. The main problem is that many therapies do not involve particularly participatory relationships, and of course, professionally trained staff are needed if the job is to be done responsibly.

Individual instruction (tutoring)

This can be a highly personal way of teaching individuals about the health issues that are relevant to them. The main advantage is that individuals get special attention. A practitioner can focus on the disease, treatment issues, and health promotion strategies relevant to each individual. Instruction does not always have to be didactic. One can tutor another person in very discursive ways, participating, in effect, in an ongoing set of conversations. This is a very good method if your health promotion work is something that involves seeing one or two individuals a week in addition to your other pastoral care or general practice duties—providing that the time you have for this function is seen as adequate on both sides. It also works well for those whose motivation is poor or fluctuating. However, this approach is time-expensive and may not be practical with groups. Unless you are employed full time to provide individual health education programs to individuals, individual instruction will simply be too time consuming for most practitioners.

Inquiry learning

One way to think about 'inquiry learning' is to view this as personal, self-directed research. Individuals formulate their own health issues and then research them. This can take place in a group or in the context of individual instruction, but the emphasis is placed on the self-development of problems, issues, or hypotheses that relate to an individual's health. This type of learning can increase motivation, but because the range of possible issues to research may be endless, evaluation of that information may be difficult. This style of learning can also be labour-intensive for both staff and participants. For the individual participant, the time involved in a personal search can also be time-consuming—but rewarding.

Lecture or discussion

This is the most traditional strategy used by educationalists of every type and is probably the easiest to execute. The educator stands or sits at the front of a room and delivers a lecture for 30, 60, or 90 minutes and invites discussion during or after the talk. Lectures can be didactic or participatory. They can be used by institutions or by individual practitioners offering health education. Lectures are an efficient way of delivering large amounts of information quickly and, if the speaker is skilled, memorably.

The main problem with lectures is that they can encourage passive learning. Clearly, however, if used with other strategies, lectures have a useful place in any broader participatory health education approach. They are, however, labour-intensive in terms of staff preparation. Lecturers must research the topic and be determined and skilled enough to deliver a lecture in an entertaining or attention-holding way. Depending on the numbers that can be expected to attend the lectures, the other problem one needs to consider is the space requirements. If particular lectures will continue to be viewed as valuable for their information (and entertainment), these can also be recorded on video tape to be used by future program participants and by those who were unable to attend because of distance or for other reasons.

Peer group discussion

'Peer group discussion' simply refers to a small group coming together for the purposes of learning. These can be reading groups or problem-solving groups or both. Groups can be flexible in their functions, and providing there are basic rules of conduct that everyone agrees to abide by, they can be powerful learning forums. Groups can also meet in a variety of settings: an institutional setting, the premises of an individual provider, or the participants' own homes. If the group sets itself clear goals, learning targets can be evaluated very well.

Programmed learning

'Programmed learning' is the technical term for methods of learning derived from teaching machines, distance educational materials, or computer programs. Basically, a written text or computer program guides the participant through a graded program of learning. Participants read a little or perform an exercise of one sort or another, then move on to answer a set of questions or to test their knowledge to see if they have learnt the basic lesson implicit in the reading or exercise.

These can be valuable, but can sometimes be too 'high-tech'. Few individuals will have access to these kinds of technology, and those institutions that might have adequate resources (for example, distance education universities) may need to design and write materials that are relevant to health promoting palliative care issues, which would involve a significant commitment of time and staff resources. Nevertheless, these technologies allow for different rates of learning and can increase motivation. On the down side, they are not social technologies, often requiring people to work alone. They are, however, easy to evaluate.

Simulations and games

This category of strategies includes role plays, case studies, socio–drama, simple games, dramatisation, and group exercises in general. Participants may act out situations in their groups as practice for similar situations in the real world; they may play games that provide insights into their own or other people's conduct or attitudes; or they may attempt simple research exercises that can teach them simple facts about the social and physical consequences of their illness or health status.

The impact of these kinds of strategies can be difficult to evaluate, particularly in the long term. Their advantage is that they are very memorable and experiential strategies. On the down side, they are not favoured by shy, reserved, or introverted people, and when deciding whether to use them in groups, one must be sensitive to individual differences in temperament.

Expert panel

Referring to it as a 'cancer panel', Greenberg (1988) suggests that practitioners invite a group of professionals from the local cancer society or hospital to speak to their groups. These professionals could be asked to provide an outline of the aetiology, detection, prevention, and therapy of cancer, and the group could then spend the remaining time asking and discussing questions raised by the talk. This provides the group with a good opportunity to ask questions of a knowledgeable group of people with whom they are not generally involved. Questions that participants may be too shy, shocked, or embarrassed to ask their own physicians might also be asked here, or this opportunity may provide them with enough conviction or curiosity to return to their doctors to ask further questions about their illnesses and treatments. The expert panel, of course, can consist of professionals who are knowledgeable about any disease, not just cancer.

The panel strategy provides a supportive environment for questions, can be easy to arrange, is highly informative, and can be arranged by institutions or individual practitioners. It is an excellent two-way feedback opportunity too, with the attending professionals learning from the participants' questions and from their responses to the professionals' knowledge and communication styles.

Directory of services

A list of professional services that are relevant to participants in health promoting palliative care is useful. Few institutions or individual practitioners are able to provide for everyone's individual needs simply because these can cover an enormous range. It is particularly important to have a list of complementary therapy services that one has personally reviewed, but be careful not to defame. It might be safer for practitioners to provide only the names of services that they endorse and to omit those they feel are substandard. It is important for participants to know that, if they should decide to use a meditation teacher or herbalist, you are at least able to provide simple information about comparative service and cost. This can be helpful to participants, and gives them a well-founded impression that there are few boundaries that a participant in health promoting palliative care can cross that place them 'outside' your orbit of care and attention.

Social strategies include:
- audiovisual aids
- counselling and behaviour modification
- individual instruction
- inquiry learning
- lectures and discussion
- peer group discussion
- programmed learning

- simulations and games
- expert panels
- a directory of services

Personal strategies

There are at least six personal strategies that one might use to encourage participants to research their self in order to clarify their values or life direction. You may think of many other ways to facilitate this kind of learning, but the examples that follow are offered as suggestions.

Memory work

This is a method that has been developed by feminist social science researchers to re-examine the social nature of personal experience. Discussions about the practical details of the method can be found in Frigga Haug (1992), Michael Schratz and Rob Walker (1995), and Glenda Koutroulis (1996). Much of what has been written has its foundation in the pioneering work of Frigga Haug.

A small group of people, perhaps not more than eight or nine, gather together to select a personal experience that is, and continues to be, important to them. It may, for example, be the time when their doctors first discussed their prognoses with them. For practitioners, it could be, for example, the events that led them to specialise in palliative nursing. Participants write down, as fully and with as much detail as possible, their memory of that experience. The story is written in the third person. The group then discusses each memory as *their* story, a story with omissions, selective recall, recurring themes, and internal contradictions and questions. The purposes of the discussion are to uncover the way that personality produces selective stories and to identify the taken-for-granted connection between social structures (for example, professional encounters or families) and personal reactions.

Since the past (or our memory of that past) helps to guide us through the present and future, one might change the present by re-considering the past. Memory work can show us how we can be drawn into conventional but sometimes unhelpful ways of thinking, which limit our choices and feelings. Other possibilities and choices might be opened up through critical group reflection. Not to be confused with therapy or encounter groups, memory work places its emphasis on the *social processes* that create the memories, rather than concentrating on the idiosyncratic nature of personal reaction alone.

Journal writing

Participants of a group can attempt to keep a personal diary or journal of their days. These could be written in the morning but concern the day before. In this way, the thoughts and activities that occurred when the person was lying or sitting awake the night before might also be recorded. The diary or journal can function as a soliloquy, which the author can analyse as if it were written by someone else. The themes that emerge in the diary can be brought to the group for discussion, and each participant can look for the common and unique elements of suffering or insight that might be derived from the journal.

Some people take to this task well, using the activity as a strategy for self-discovery but also as a way of 'ventilating' or 'unloading' on paper. Like a magic trick, a person can put the day's stresses away, dumping them onto the pages, closing the book, and then reading them the next day as though they are strange things that happened to someone else. Others find it difficult to write, but should be encouraged to write or perhaps tape-record their 'journal' of their daily journey into the experience of living with serious illness. The medium itself is not important. The messages that each person might excavate from them later may, however, be very important for that person down the track.

Letter writing

Letter writing is similar to journal writing, but is not necessarily a daily exercise. Like memory work, it can be an activity that is used to examine a particular issue that is important to an individual. Perhaps there are things individuals would like to say to their doctors but feel that, for one reason or another, they cannot. Perhaps there are some things that practitioners would like to say to particular patients but cannot. Instead they can write a letter to the relevant person and, rather than sending it, take it to their group to discuss it with other group members.

This sort of letter writing (the unsent letter) has five important functions according to Schratz and Walker (1995, pp. 137–45). Letters provide private space for personal communication. You can express some things better alone than when you are face to face with others or in front of authority figures. And the mere act of expressing them might be important for you. Second, letters are located in time, meaning that they can show the progress of a relationship or experience or change. Letters are forms of communication that allow you to choose the right time—the time when you are in the right mood. A letter is also a medium that allows you to exercise control over the presentation of self. Finally, letters can be important sources of feedback for the self (on subsequent re-reading), for others (if you decide to send or speak them), and for the group (as one form of communication *to* them).

Vox populi

Aside from writing, individuals might also use tape recordings to examine issues important to them. Groups can decide on a series of questions that a person should provide thoughtful answers to, and these might be recorded rather than written. Hand-held tapes are useful for these kinds of tasks. This strategy is particular useful for people who are not comfortable with writing.

Vox populi was originally designed as a method that attempted to capture people's daily experiences as they occurred. An interviewer would regularly record a person's daily experience at the car plant or the offices of IBM or at the check-out counter of a local supermarket. But these are records that you can keep for yourself too. Regularly recording your experiences, day and night, for a typical week can help you to see how that experience *is* for you or how you are telling yourself about that experience. You can later analyse these records as a kind of 'data' source that helps you to understand your own experience.

Perceptual maps

A strategy that is perhaps less trouble and may be quicker than self-taping or writing is for individuals to draw maps or pictorial representations of their current life experiences. They might draw their favourite foods. Or they could pictorially chart their physical exercise histories or their relationships with their doctors or families. Some people are more comfortable with this form of expression than with spoken or written forms. After discussing the themes or other features of the drawings, individuals might then re-draw them to represent the new insights they have gained from studying the old drawings. On the other hand, they might speculate about the other ways they might have been able to draw the scenes and rate the probability of those drawings becoming a reality for them.

Photograph album or life story

Aside from reflecting on critical events and experiences in life, and going beyond the importance of scrutinising daily or weekly events, it can be important to reflect broadly on the kinds of people we are or have become. This is not, and should not be, an exercise in personality exploration as might be conducted in therapeutic contexts, but rather it is an exploration of the assemblage of social, personal, and spiritual values that make us the 'characters' that we are (Kellehear 1993, pp. 74–81). You can borrow or purchase an empty photo album and fill it with old photos that allow you to tell the story of your self as you now understand it. Like all memory work, this will necessarily involve omissions and biases, but it can be a good starting point for understanding the importance of your own honest reflection at this time, and it permits a certain flexible and critical insight into how precarious your self-image is.

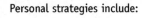

Personal strategies include:

- memory work
- journal writing
- letter writing
- vox populi
- perceptual maps
- photo album or life story

A MEMORY, A DREAM, AND A REFLECTION

There are three observations to take away from this chapter on health education. First, remember that the strategies that are employed in health education will often be the same strategies that are used when exploring issues about death, dying, and grief. The processes of education about health are underpinned by the same assumptions and ideals that inform education about death.

Second, the strategies used in the health education field result from a combination of experience and creative thinking about learning. Many of the strategies were derived from the experience of working in schools, in workplaces, or in other cultures or social classes with a dream to improve health in those places. There is, however, nothing particularly valuable about them in themselves. The strategies have value only insofar as they have worth to those who work with the seriously ill. Pick, choose, experiment, disregard, dispose, and invent strategies as you need to. We all need to start somewhere. This chapter is as good a place to start your thinking as any.

Finally, the driving values behind the health education expressions of a health promoting palliative care are participation, respect for social and professional differences, and critical self-reflection. In other words, the aims of health education in health promoting palliative care are to listen and facilitate, to promote social and professional tolerance for different viewpoints, and to encourage research into self and the health issues important to that self.

4

Death Education

Men fear death,

as children fear to go in the dark;

and as that natural fear in children is increased

   with tales,

so is the other.

Francis Bacon, as quoted in Selby 1912, p. 3

The simple aim of any death education program is to encourage people to learn what they need to know about death and dying. Most of this death education, most of its history, and most of the books and articles on this subject are targeted at students and professionals. This is certainly true of death education in the USA (see Pine 1986).

This chapter is principally concerned with death education for those who are living with a serious illness and where the prospect of death is an equally serious possibility. However, there are many reasons why death education is important for *all* people, and not just those with terminal or life-threatening illness.

First, we must ask the question 'Why not death education for all?' Nothing is more certain than death. Furthermore, most of us will encounter the death of others during the course of our lifetimes—the longer we live, the more experience we will have of death. Experience shows that these are difficult social and emotional times for everyone. The failure to make at least minor preparations for these events and experiences seems to be a tad remiss, to say the least. Preparation for disasters such as cyclones or building fires, which are merely possible, is seen as sensible and responsible. So how much more rational are preparations for a 'dead' certainty such as death itself?

Second, many people fear death. It is not true that people fear the unknown—a contradiction in terms—but people do fill the unknown with particular fears that they associate with death. They may fear a painful death. They may fear a lack of control over their material affairs. They may fear life after death—or no life after death. People may express anxiety about the fortunes and welfare of those they are leaving behind. Death education can help in alleviating some of these anxieties.

Third, death education can assist in preparing people—psychologically and socially—for the prospect of death. In this context, people are able to identify and take practical steps to get their material affairs in order.

Fourth, death education can simply reduce ignorance about death—its practical issues or its religious and spiritual connections—thereby helping to reduce the prospect of equally ignorant, and potentially troublesome, responses to death and dying.

Finally, death education can assist in clarifying values (Eddy & Duff 1986). Where people have not even thought about death itself until it finally demonstrates its undeniable presence, death education can facilitate a strong, renewed, and highly focused reflection and clarification of their own views and values. This education may have important and obvious benefits in the clarification of life values in general and may have practical implications for how people may live during their remaining time.

The various strategies and processes for death education are broadly similar to those already identified in the previous chapter on health education. We need not go over that ground. Instead, in this chapter, we will cover the four most important content areas to be covered in any death education program for those with life-threatening or terminal illness, beginning with broad topics of relevance to the theme of death and human experience. We will then look at social legacy (that is, issues relevant to 'settling one's affairs'). In looking at life after death, we will touch on the eschatological issue of whether human beings survive death. Finally, we will look at loss and grief, focusing on how to discuss the social and personal issues relating to loss (as opposed to the therapeutic issues).

Important topic areas for death education:
- death and human experience
- social legacy
- life beyond death
- loss and grief

DEATH AND HUMAN EXPERIENCE

It may be desirable to begin a discussion and learning opportunity about death with a general survey or reflection about death and human experience. It might be easier and gentler to begin with an impersonal introduction to death and dying issues and then gradually to move the discussion to more personal concerns.

The 'design' or 'curriculum' that one might use to peruse the general field of death and human experience will be up to your group or the individual client to decide, but you might think about a list of topics such as:

- the history of our ideas about death
- media portrayals of death
- death portrayed by the giants of philosophy and art
- music and poetry about death, the afterlife, grief and bereavement, euthanasia, or dying

You might combine some of these topics and begin with a short history of death and dying in the Western world, move to the portrayal of these ideas in music, art, poetry, and literature, and end with contemporary ideas as these are found in media such as television, radio, film, and newspapers. The ideas about death found within Christianity or other world religions could also be an interesting topic to explore here. There are several valuable resources that one might use for this introduction.

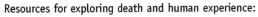

Resources for exploring death and human experience:
- popular books
- films
- music
- art
- philosophical works

Popular books

There is a major genre of books that ponder the meaning of death. You may already know many yourself. The following are only examples of that genre: Leo Tolstoy's (1960) *The Death of Ivan Ilyich*; Alexander

Solzhenitsyn's (1968) *Cancer Ward*; Evelyn Waugh's (1948) *The Loved One*; Robert Dessaix's (1996) *Night Letters*; Gillian Rose's (1995) philosophically reflective *Love's Work*; Lily Pincus's (1976) *Death and the Family*; and Albert Camus's (1961) *The Outsider*. Each of these books provides reflections on death either from the perspective of certain personalities or characters who are central to the book's story line or from the personal perspective of the author.

More abstract, perhaps, but no less useful are a number of general works that take a broader approach to death, people, and history: *The Oxford Book of Death* (Enright 1987); Bert Keizer's (1996) *Dancing with Mr D*; F. Birrell and F. L. Lucas's (1930) *The Art of Dying: An Anthology* (compiling famous last words); Michael Kearl's (1989) academic but accessible book *Endings*; and Jessica Mitford's (1980) old but still provocative and evocative book *The American Way of Death*. Another old but interesting volume is Virginia Moore's (1946) *Ho for Heaven! Man's Changing Attitude toward Dying*. A more scholarly but no less interesting volume by a famous French historian is Phillipe Aries (1974) *Western Attitudes toward Death*.

Kathy Charmaz and colleagues' (1997) book *The Unknown Country: Death in Australia, Britain, and the USA* is also a useful historical introduction to major Western social influences on reactions to death. You may also wish to take a dispassionate and unsparing look at the process of death itself by reading Sherwin Nuland's (1994) *How We Die*. Remember when reading Nuland's book that the description of an experience by an outsider to that experience, no matter how graphic, is often quite different from that experience as told by the experiencer. Nuland describes death, however carefully, as an outsider.

In a more reflective vein, some very good examples of explorations of the meaning of death by 'outsiders' can be found in volumes such as Caroline Jones's (1989) *The Search for Meaning*, and Rosemary Dinnage's (1992) *The Ruffian on the Stair: Reflections on Death*. Savary and O'Connor's (1973) *The Heart Has its Seasons* is also a worthy addition to any library, providing a reflective resource on life, death, and beyond. And other valuable and highly readable volumes are Elizabeth Kubler-Ross's (1978) *To Live until We Say Good-bye* and Victor Frankel's (1973) *The Doctor and the Soul* (especially the chapter 'On the Meaning of Death').

Films

There is also a long history of cinematic portrayals and meditations on the subject of death. Often, of course, death is used as a secondary theme in order to explore other themes such as friendship, romantic love, or parental relations. *The Shadow Box*, *Love Story*, *Steel Magnolias*, *Sunshine*, and *Terms of Endearment* are examples of films that perform these kinds of functions and explore these types of themes.

Other films, such as *Death takes a Holiday*, directly examine our existential relationship with death. This film explores the idea of what would happen if there were no death. In the film, death does take a few days away from his (yes, death is a man) normal duties to see what all the fuss is about. In the meantime, sick and dying people are unable to die. Death visits a boarding house where he engages people in a discussion about why people fear him. Fascinating viewing.

Another instructive piece of viewing is to compare the British film *Truly, Madly, Deeply* with the American film *Ghost*. Both films are about the death of a partner, but shortly after this death, each of the surviving partners in their respective films is 'visited' by the dead partner. Both films are instructive both as symbolic explorations of grief and bereavement and as culture-specific cinematic portrayals of life after death for the dead and for the survivors at a time when popular culture is renewing its interest in ghosts, visions of the bereaved, and life after death.

Music

Richard Pacholski (1986a), and Charles Lochner and Robert Stevenson (1988) provide a useful introduction to the possibilities of death education that employs music. Lochner and Stevenson provide an introduction to how they use music to help the dying and bereaved. This is yet another genre of literature on the subject. Those interested in music 'therapy' for dying and bereaved people have written their own books on the subject and also contribute regular articles in journals such as the *Journal of Music Therapy*.

Pacholski (1986a) provides an early but still very useful discussion of bibliographic sources on the subject of music as a prompt for contemplation about death and dying. The style of such musical prompts ranges from blues, rock and roll, and folk music to opera, hymns, and requiem music. The music of mourning is particularly interesting, and he identifies styles such as apotheoses (works written in honour of the dead), deplorations (mourning poems or songs), dirges (laments, or funeral or burial hymns), elegies (more laments), or epicidiums (music expressing grief), among many others. The world of lament and loss as expressed in music is explored by this author in a fascinating and witty manner, and this article is definitely worth the attention of those who wish to employ music as an important or passing component of their death education programs.

Art

What Pacholski does for musicology bibliographies he also does for the visual arts (1986b). He lists 154 bibliographic sources that might be useful for those wishing to employ art as a general introduction to the theme of death. This bibliography is a good starting point for novices in this area, and it would be useful to examine it *before* requesting a general bibliographic search at your local library. Pacholski's work will allow you to understand the parameters of any search, and will prompt you to think in more specific terms about how you want to approach this complex area.

Philosophical works

There are some good books that provide a broad overview of the 'problem' of death, and many of these are considered 'classics' in their respective fields. The following are what I consider to be the most readable ones.

If you can relate to the idea that human nature incorporates life and death instincts that pull and push our lives and desires in different directions, then Sigmund Freud's (1971) *Beyond the Pleasure Principle* might be a good read. (Also see Freud's (1915) 'Thoughts for the Times on War and Death', to be found in his collected works, edited by J. Strachey.) And while we are mentioning psychoanalytic views, we should also remember Norman O. Brown's (1968) *Life against Death: The Psychoanalytic Meaning of History*, and similarly Ernest Becker's (1973) Pulitzer Prize winning *The Denial of Death*.

Gil Elliot's (1972) journalistic but thought-provoking *Twentieth Century Book of the Dead* reminds us of the material and historical context in which death has occurred over the last one hundred years. On a more spiritual note, John Hick's (1976) *Death and Eternal Life* takes us on a tour of the world's religions. He attempts to evaluate how much of these ideas we might legitimately employ to form a fair impression of our prospects beyond the grave. Finally, a more interdisciplinary and reflective approach is taken by Darryl Reanney (1994) in *Music of the Mind*. Reanney takes us on a wild ride through physics, philosophy, and psychology to look at the fate of the human spirit—a disturbing, thought-provoking, and enlightening work.

SOCIAL LEGACY

The first and most obvious area of personal interest in death education will probably involve issues to do with the need to 'settle one's affairs'. In other words, it is important that people are encouraged at least to think about the things (both material and social) that they want to give to other people before they die or leave to them after their death. It is useful to learn about social legacy.

There are four relevant areas to any death education that considers legacy issues.

Social legacy issues include:
- material preparations for death
- adjusting others for one's possible absence
- farewells and personal legacies
- provisions for animal companions (pets)

Material preparations for death

Outside the USA, where will-making is popular and taken for granted, there are significant numbers of people who are intestate—that is, they do not possess a will. The will, as a legal document, is not particularly complex, and proformas, for example, can be bought in many non-legal outlets such as newsagents or accountancy firms. Some people feel insecure about following the instructions on these do-it-yourself wills and prefer to obtain legal advice. That advice is usually inexpensive, but a short visit by a legal or financial counsellor might be a useful part of any educational program dealing with such preparations.

General issues to do with financial status and provisions for survivors raise similar concerns. A person's financial situation may not be complex, perhaps extending to several bank accounts and a pension fund (sometimes also called a 'superannuation fund'). Nevertheless, considerable anxiety can be generated over even these issues, and some people become concerned about the possible expense of obtaining financial advice. A guest speaker can provide an informal opportunity to discuss the range of fees and benefits available to people.

Other people might be interested in prepaid funeral arrangements or may have particular wishes in relation to personalising their funerals but are unsure of prices or how to make such arrangements. Most people have never even spoken to anyone at their local funeral company about such issues. It can be useful to provide this kind of information in the form of brochures about products, services, options, and contact phone numbers for further enquiries. For some people, dealing with this kind of information can be less stressful than making such enquiries on the premises of these establishments.

Many people also have an interest in donating parts or the whole of their bodies to 'science'. This is not always appropriate for people who die of an advanced malignancy or HIV/AIDS, but it can be useful to explore the issues of if, how, and when this option might be possible, and for whom. Again, a medical visitor to a health promoting program could give valuable advice about this. It also might usefully be integrated into a broader health education discussion.

Several useful books have been published about settling one's affairs in order, and some of these could be useful to have on site for convenient general perusal (see Anderson 1991).

Adjusting others for one's possible absence

In an early social study of terminally ill people's conduct (Kellehear 1990), I found a significant number of people who were concerned about preparing people for their absence. These were mainly, but not exclusively, women. Among the top concerns were:

- the remarriage of their spouses
- the fact that some of their children, particularly younger children, might grow up without really knowing who they were or what they were really like
- resolving long-standing family or friendship tensions and conflict
- minimising the financial impact of their future absence on their spouses or children

More than a few of these people found these concerns difficult to confront, but were convinced and committed to dealing with them in one form or another. This has two implications for any death education program. First, these issues are valuable topics for group discussion. Support, empathy, and creative ideas can be the result of discussing these issues as 'the group's' general concern. Problem-solving within the group may provide particular individuals with ideas, support, or confidence in personally approaching the relevant people with whom they so dearly want to resolve things.

Second, when personal approaches are too difficult, fraught, or unsuccessful, other options for individuals may be possible, but these need to be identified and the resource or process issues explained. In this context, the producing of audiovisual material, the writing of letters, and the arrangement of gifts at important times could all or separately be important options. It may be useful to share drafts of letters. The process involved in making a video message may need explanation and a little technical training. A gift and its timing may need some thought. These are important tasks within a death education program that is both personal and relevant.

Farewells and personal legacies

Dying is about leaving. We go somewhere, whether it is some biblical 'heaven', a spiritualist summer land, or into the chain of physical processes that make up the universe as we know it. Before leaving anything, it is customary and polite to bid farewell, and that is precisely what most people—not all, but most people—want (Kellehear 1990, pp. 157–69). The only real questions are when, how, and to whom one directs the farewells. Therefore, discussion of the nature and timing of farewells is part of a useful death education program.

Some people wish to say goodbye when they are well and ambulant. Some of these people do not wish the occasion to be obvious to the person to whom they are 'saying goodbye'. Others want a party every bit as cheerful as their twenty-first birthday or wedding reception. Yet others want their farewells to be 'deathbed' farewells and may need the cooperation and help of hospice staff. And other people do not wish to make a verbal farewell but would rather use a video or letter, even a gift, for the purposes.

A few people find the idea of saying goodbyes not only threatening to their idea of hope and interpersonal stability, but also personally irksome in the face of serious illness. There are no 'correct' ways to die. The cultural defines or shapes the personal, and a useful death education is one that not only facilitates practical processes of social legacy, such as saying goodbye, but also helps those who have other preferences to clarify their values thoughtfully.

Finally, a lot of people ask a more existential question about their legacy: what will I, as an individual, leave behind me as a contribution to life? This is another way of asking 'What was the purpose of my life? If and when I leave this life, what will my personal legacy to others be?' This is a useful task, and many people ask themselves this question when their minds turn to the issue of legacy. Many people do not simply see this issue in material terms. Some will see their legacy in terms of their children, or their life's work, or the role they have played in service clubs and organisations. Others may see their legacy in terms of whether they will 'leave' the place better than it was when they 'arrived'. These are difficult, often quite disturbing questions. If you do not believe me, stop for a moment and ask yourself these questions right now.

I met a woman once who believed that she had lived a 'very ordinary life'. After reflection, she came to the belief that her legacy was the love of people that she had shown consistently through life. As a symbol of this legacy, she determined that she would make dolls to give away to as many people as she could before she died. During the course of her illness, which spanned only a year, she made over seventy dolls for her friends and hospital staff. The dolls, and what they meant to her, were her legacy—what she would leave to others.

An exploration of 'what my life might mean in positive terms to others' can be useful as a discussion topic or as a private written or diary-type exercise. The question, and its answer, can be vital to peace of mind and, therefore, too important to ignore in any death education process for those facing death, or even those who are not.

Provisions for animal companions

People are not the only ones left behind when a person dies. Most people own animal companions, usually a dog or cat or three. Despite a tendency in some social quarters to trivialise human–pet relations, the reality is that animal companions are very important relationships for many people (see Katcher & Beck 1983; Sussman 1985; Lee & Lee 1992, Kellehear & Fook 1997).

Buried in a collection of stories that are a tribute to Australian working dogs (Goode 1992, pp. 34–8) lies a poignant story by Geoffrey Blight of Narrogin in Western Australia. 'Happy Father's Day' tells the story of a farmer with terminal cancer and his relationship with his working dog, 'Rusty', during the farmer's last few weeks of life:

> Nothing whatsoever was said between man and dog. At the hospital entrance I lifted dad into the wheelchair. He stared straight ahead. No words, not even a glance at Rusty. As I moved the chair back to shut the car door, the old dog sat, nose pressed hard against the glass. Still the man stared ahead, now visibly upset and trembling,
>
> For a moment I thought I might say something but could not. As I started to push the chair away an old hand suddenly came out and bony old fingers pressed hard against the glass. Their eyes met for the last time and in a moment not meant for me, the old man, tears streaming freely down his cheeks, mumbled, 'Goodbye, old boy,' and we moved slowly away (Blight in Goode 1992, p. 37).

This story, like so many thousands of similar published and oral accounts, highlights the importance of animals for rural dwellers and suburban families alike. But it is in the literature on pets rather than the literature on palliative care that we find a significant discussion of these experiences. The companion animal is rendered invisible in most discourses about health care.

Provision for the care of animals, even the existence of these animals, should not be overlooked or taken for granted. Not everyone has someone to care for their animals or knows a circle of people who they would trust to care for their pet. And some people are embarrassed to raise these issues for fear of ridicule. Other people feel that euthanasia for their animals is their only choice—a choice that is as traumatic for some as the prospect of their own deaths. Discussion of the options and enquiries to local vets, the relevant animal protection society, and/or dog homes might be important sources of information, social networks for adopting out, and support services. Some people fear that illness or death may separate them from their pets before adequate provisions are made, and this fear might be addressed as a normal part of any death education program.

It goes without saying that most of these issues benefit from being shared in group situations. However, if your health promoting palliative care program is largely a one-to-one affair, then it will be important to be sensitive to these areas. A questioning approach is not the most useful strategy either. Sometimes it might be easier for people to discuss their concerns about legacy if you are able to disclose your own concerns in these areas. Alternatively, you may sympathetically relate stories of other people for whom these legacy concerns were important.

LIFE BEYOND DEATH

'Life after death' is a controversial topic these days. Gone are the days when you could take it for granted that everybody believed that one survived bodily death because the 'soul' joined God in Heaven or the Devil in Hell. Furthermore, even though there are sizeable numbers of people who still believe that this scenario is likely, a significant number of people are not so sure these days.

Many people, particularly the well educated from professional classes (Gallop 1982), doubt that human survival over death is possible at all. Many of these people now believe that life begins, is solely associated with material embodiment, and dies when the body itself dies. There is no life beyond death. What attitude might a health promoting palliative care worker take to all this?

There is one fundamental issue that does not change, despite our changing attitudes to the problem of human survival after death, and it is useful to remind ourselves of this before proceeding on this topic. The basic reality is this: there is no 'proof' that we do, or do not, survive death. Evidence exists to support both sides of the debate. At the base of the different arguments, there are important philosophical assumptions and differences, and these go largely unrecognised.

Those who believe that human beings survive death (believers, religionists, New Agers, dualists, and so on) believe that there is a part of a person that survives the death of the body (the soul, astral body, spirit, and so on). This part goes on to 'another world', where it continues to have a full and interesting life for better or worse, depending on the belief system and moral characteristics of the person in question. These kinds of believers are often greatly impressed with stories of personal testimony—stories about near-death experiences, clairvoyance, or extra-sensory perception (ESP) for example.

Those who believe that we die with the body and nothing survives (materialists, monists, sceptics, epiphenomenalists, and so on) believe that there is nothing to life beyond the physical processes that support our daily consciousness. They are often cast in the role of critics of those who believe in survival, but in reality both sides are 'believers' because no final evidence has settled the debate. Sceptical people are often greatly impressed by neurophysiological explanations about the brain and its workings.

Nothing much changes in the cultures from which the respective arguments emanate, each being impressed with its own arguments and cleverness. Each year produces new books on how the brain works and that bravely declare that dualism is dead (the idea that people have a 'mind' separate from the 'body' and that the former is not necessarily dependent on the latter). With less fanfare, but with usually higher sales, other books will appear regaling readers with stories of how people have 'died' and come back to us to tell us 'there is no death'. And although many sceptical readers are likely to be irritated (rather than seriously persuaded), these stories will mention some incident that 'cannot be explained' by current 'medical science'. The academic and media debates are stirred up again and the next round of tail-chasing begins.

At the end of the day, it is up to each one of us to make up his or her own mind about what is, or is not, convincing, and the work of death education should be to ensure that people are familiar with:

1 the basic experiences that are considered to be compelling evidence of survival
2 some of the basic objections

In that spirit, then, the following sections are designed to provide a quick overview of some important topic areas and of individual references that I have found to be helpful introductions to them. Of course, there is so much literature in the area, and everyone has their 'favourites', so if you know this literature well, you may prefer other selections.

General introductions

One of the first descriptions of a death education program that took 'life beyond death' as its central theme was of a course developed by V. Q. Wacks (1988). Wacks outlines his lecture topics and some of his readings for a course in eschatology (a study of the afterlife or final resting state of the soul). However, unlike Wacks, my references are for health promotion workers rather than for clients. This does not mean that these references are not relevant for clients. However, the decision to use them in whole or part, to relay that information orally in discussion or as photocopied readings, or to use them in any other form is a decision that will vary from program to program, and my discussion of them should not be seen to favour any one of these options.

Good general introductions to Christian arguments about the life beyond can be gleaned from the Protestant writer John Hick in his *Death and Eternal Life* (1976) and the Catholic writer Hans Kung (1984) in *Eternal Life?* A quick review of concepts of the afterlife in world religions, especially non-Christian religions, can be gleaned from Dan Cohn-Sherbock and Christopher Lewis's (1995) *Beyond Death*. A most interesting review of how present concepts of the after-life grew out of our evolving contemplation of this problem over the centuries is gained from Colleen McDannell and Bernhard Lang's (1988) *Heaven: A History*.

Near-death experiences

Near-death experiences, as I am sure most people are now aware, are experiences of crisis brought about by serious injury or medical emergency. People report that, while they were unconscious, they 'left their bodies', met deceased or supernatural beings, and perhaps experienced a review of their lives. Other reports include the sensation of being drawn into a dark tunnel, feelings of euphoria and great happiness, and sighting beautiful cities and communities populated by people who had long been dead.

When beginning an examination of near-death experiences, you cannot go past the accessible and eternally popular 'first' work on the subject by Raymond Moody (1975), *Life after Life*, and Ken Ring's (1980) follow-up, but more systematic, work *Life at Death*. A more scholarly and historical treatment of the subject is provided in Carol Zaleski's (1987) *Otherworld Journeys*. For some critical analyses of near-death experiences and the studies that report them, you might consult Susan Blackmore's (1993) *Dying to Live* and my own (1996) *Experiences Near Death*.

Related to the literature on near-death experiences is the literature on near-death visions. Studies of doctors and nurses who have sat with dying people reveal that a significant proportion of those dying report visions that include reunions with former friends and relatives who have previously died. The best-selling work in this genre of literature is Karliss Osis and Erlendur Haraldsson's (1977) *At the Hour of our Death*. The critical remarks about the literature on near-death experiences equally apply to this genre of work.

Mediumship/electronic voice phenomena

There is a large literature on mediumship and the related phenomenon called 'channelling'. Mediumship is popular with spiritualists. They believe that they are able to communicate with the dead through certain 'gifted' people who are able, sometimes in a trance state, to communicate telepathically with those 'gone before us'. Accusations of fraud and deception are standard here, and it is difficult for a reasonable person not to be impressed by the corruption that has dogged this area. Beyond the obvious frauds, however, are those mediums who do seem to possess knowledge only known to individuals or those close to individuals (such as their dead friends and relatives). In these cases, the charge is that mediumistic messages are vague, made to fit the multiple interpretations of those who are eager to be convinced of contact and who are tricked into inadvertently supplying information by succumbing to leading questions. For mediums and their messages, any theosophical book store and many New Age booksellers will supply all the information and references that you need. For a sceptical view of the revival of interest in this area, you might look at Richard Basil's (1989) very witty and well-researched *Not Necessarily the New Age*.

You do not, however, need a human medium to receive messages from 'the other side'. A simple tape recorder switched on and left for a few minutes at a time will, with persistence on your part, produce 'voices' that will address you. This is called Raudive Voice Phenomena (after one of the original researchers, Konstantin Raudive) or more generally Electronic Voice Phenomena (EVP).

Good introductions to the subject are Raudive's (1971) *Breakthrough*, Bill Welch's (1975) *Talks with the Dead*, and an account of the honestly compelling experiment conducted by the interested British journalist Peter Bander (1973). A critical account of this phenomenon can be gleaned from David Ellis's (1978) *The Mediumship of the Tape Recorder*. It seems that the voices can be quite hard to hear, particularly at first. Some of the voices may in fact be radio waves accidentally garbled onto magnetic tape. Although no one disputes that voices appear on the tapes, the '$5000-dollar question' is: are they the voices of the dead?

Visions of the bereaved

A lot of people who have lost children or spouses to death have reported subsequent 'contact' with them. Sometimes, these people report hearing former relatives' or friends' voices talking to them. At other times, a fully embodied appearance takes place before their very eyes. Many of these accounts can be found in a popular United States book by the Guggenheims (1996) called *Hello from Heaven* and in Louis LaGrand's (1997) more analytical but no less compelling *After Death Communication*. Raymond Moody (1993), of near-death experiences fame, claims that he is able to induce such experiences with the help of relaxation techniques, a mirror, and a dark room. Believe it or not. His book is aptly entitled *Reunions*. A critical account of spontaneous appearances of the dead can be found in R. C. Finucane's (1996) fascinating and equally well-titled account *Ghosts*.

Appearances of the dead seem to follow a pattern that is predictably social, and their messages, far from being revealing, are often quite banal. This has been another criticism of mediumistic messages. But postcards from friends on holiday are often banal too, but I don't disbelieve that they are on holiday because of that. For instance, when a lucky friend of mine visited Nice on the Cote d'Azur several years ago, I had never been to such an exciting place. What information did I get when she finally arrived at that famous location? What wonders did I learn from her short but kind communication from that faraway and romantic place?

> Dear Allan and Jan: It's a dog's life here no doubt. They're everywhere. The local shop selling diamante collars is called Aristochien! We found a Greek restaurant. Very warm. That tube station is Chancery Lane. See you soon. Jeanne.

Well, the sceptics might ask if that is the best Jeanne can do. Unfortunately, the answer must be that yes, apparently it is. Her message could be considered banal, but I was lucky to get a postcard at all given the good time she was having. I do not know what 'very warm' means either—it could refer to the restaurant, or it could be describing the weather. The comment about Chancery Lane is, I think, a reminder about a rail station in London that I had forgotten during an earlier conversation on a topic that I can no longer remember. All this banality, forgetfulness, and brevity, and we are only talking about France— not the afterlife! The study of life beyond death in the course of any death education program should be approached with some openness and humility.

LOSS AND GRIEF

One of the perennial topics in palliative care is that of loss and grief. But in the context of a health promoting palliative care, which is a set of strategies based on a social model of care, the primary task is to encourage people to view loss and grief as *normal* and *regularly occurring* human experiences. It is not the responsibility of health promotion workers to supply 'therapeutic' responses to people with grief. This is the proper work of those whose experience and expertise lies in grief work. For people whose sense of loss and grief is great and burden-some, a referral to these services might be relevant and useful. But in the context of death education, it is useful to make two observations.

First, many models of grief are culture-specific and often cannot be applied across different social classes, ethnic groups, or ages (Walter 1997). The commonly accepted American model of grief, which encourages people to 'ventilate' and express their grief, may not suit everyone.

Related to this observation is the second, more individual applica-tion of this principle, which is that many people remain committed to the private view that the rigours of personal sorrow should not be shared with others. Some people prefer to grieve alone and in private. This does not mean, however, that the same people would not posi-tively seek to discuss their grief with others, and/or benefit from sharing their experiences with others in similar situations. Nor does this necessarily mean that *some* personal sorrow is not shared. It can mean, instead, that many people do not necessarily desire to have their 'grief' problematised or analysed by professional contact unless they are having special difficulties in coping with this experience. They will not necessarily know if they are experiencing 'special difficulties' unless they know from past experience, other people's experience, or the rel-evant literature what is 'usual' or 'normal' about those experiences.

Exchanges, readings, or discussions that are shared in a casual and friendly atmosphere are often useful first responses to loss and grief, are often most welcome, and are relevant to any death education that pro-motes health. A group reflection or extended discussion about loss and grief in everyday contexts, therefore, will be an important topic to include in a health promoting palliative care program.

I am regularly reminded of the interesting United States study (Carpenter 1977) that asked people the simple question of what they used their screwdrivers for. Most people answered that they used their screwdrivers to turn screws, and that this was not a regular task for them. They rarely used their humble carpentry tool. But when the researchers asked to see the actual screwdriver, and the tool was physically inspected, all the parties—interviewers and interviewees alike—realised something quite telling. The screwdriver played a much bigger part in people's lives than most people remembered or thought possible. People used screwdrivers as hammers, digging instruments, stirrers of liquids as diverse as house paint and coffee. Other people had used their screwdrivers as miniature jemmies to pry open jammed windows or doors, car boots, or troublesome jam jars. Initially these stories were prompted by the interviewers asking the owners for explanations about paint or chip marks on the screwdrivers, or about why the tools were bent, twisted, or blunt, but then other stories emerged quickly, which the physical appearance of the tool did not originally suggest. There was the time when the screwdriver was used as a temporary tent peg, as a 'weapon' between a warring brother and sister, or as a toy—a throwing dart or knife—on a boring summer's afternoon while idly talking to friends. There was another time when the tool acted as a convenient (if shameful) instrument to turn the steak on the barbecue when, in a billow of smoking meat, its owner couldn't find the barbecue tongs. And the stories rolled on.

The theme of this story, or set of stories, is that much of our life and its little experiences are taken-for-granted. Loss and grief are some of those taken-for-granted experiences that it can be beneficial to stop and recall. Jobs, travel, relationships, hopes and dreams, marriages, promotions, stages of life such as youth or the teenage years—all of these, for many people, entail experiences of loss and perhaps not a little grief. What were our feelings then? What personal lessons, if any, did we draw from those times, either at the time or later? What became of those feelings and thoughts, and how have those experiences evolved up to now? What do you make of them now? How, if at all, do they relate to your current situation and experience? And in all the experiences of change in a person's life, perhaps some of the most difficult are those related to death. Sometimes this will be the death of parents, a child, a friend, or a spouse. In later life there are hardly any people who have not experienced these kinds of loss and been brought, through the experience, to reflect on their own mortality.

And finally, be careful not to identify death education too literally with topics about death. There are other topics that are not literally about death but that may point to it in indirect ways, and some of these might usefully be raised and discussed. One topic that might fit this category is the fear that some people may hold about 'reoccurrence' of symptoms or, if they are in remission, the return of the cancer. It might be useful to explore what a return of the disease or to ill health might mean to people, and to examine whether this relates to a fear of death or to the grief about the loss of a former ideal self.

SOME FINAL REFLECTIONS

Taking some time out to stop and reflect on the nature of death and one's own appointment with this event can be useful for everyone. Doing this with others can be highly informative because of the sharing of both information and experience. This is the simple nature of any good death education.

In chapter 3 I have emphasised the importance of the participatory process involved in this learning, and in this chapter I have suggested topic areas that have been traditionally important to people confronting death. There may be other topics not discussed here that you may think, or your client group may think, are equally important. Furthermore, you should not read too much into the order in which I have discussed these topics. It may be that the discussion of loss and grief issues could be an important introduction to a general interest in the theme of death in history, music or literature. For some individuals, the topics of death in history or art may be too abstract and middle class, and many people will prefer instead to cut to more interesting topics, such as life beyond death or perhaps the technical details of how to arrange their finances. The order and priority of topics are not, in themselves, important. This chapter has served as a way of signalling some of the topics that might be valuable to discuss with people.

Finally, one should be aware of different ethnic values with respect to discussing death or dying. People from some ethnic groups—for example, people from Greece, Japan, or China—are uncomfortable talking about these topics. For some of these people, frank discussions about death can be 'bad luck', offensive, or highly threatening. To be sensitive to these possibilities, you need to make all participants aware of the weekly topics *before* their attendance. This provides people with an opportunity to discuss their reservations with you or to avoid sessions that give offence or are unhelpful to them. If your death education sessions are one-on-one sessions with individuals, you need to be aware of this possibility and of the cultural diversity of those who you serve, and adapt your approach accordingly.

On the other hand, you may be from a specific cultural background and be serving only those with that background. You will, in that instance, automatically modify the death education approach to suit your particular cultural requirements. This is an important ethical consideration in the provision of death education, because not everyone is 'empowered' by an 'open' awareness and frank discussion of death and dying issues. At the very least, some people prefer a more subtle exploration of these issues that complements and respects their individual cultural prohibitions and prescriptions.

The important lesson of this chapter, however, is that death education along some of the lines outlined in this chapter is an essential and constructive part of health promotion for most people with life-threatening or terminal illness. This is because such reflections and education can be important to all people. For those with serious illness, however, death education may help promote a further sense of control and perhaps lessen some of the anxiety that surrounds the subject of death.

5

Social Supports

But Mary kept all these things, pondering them in
her heart.

Luke 2:19

The primary function of any health promoting palliative care program is to provide support—in the form of information, education, advocacy, referral, but also small group, interpersonal support. Clearly, strategies for social support must come from a diverse and varied set of sources. They must emerge from the everyday worlds of family, workplace, and church. Ideally, they should also be contained in the sounds and visual images that emanate from television, film, radio, or the daily newspapers.

A health promoting palliative care that is concerned with the whole array of social supports in the community should be concerned not only with the reorientation of mainstream health services and attitudes to living with dying, but also with the non-health-system sources of support. These are sometimes referred to as the 'structural' or wider system issues underlying social support.

This is the first of two chapters concerned with these issues of social support. Here, I will describe and examine the issues relevant to the direct provision of small group, interpersonal support. In chapter 7, I will review possibilities and strategies for the indirect encouragement and enhancement of wider support for people living with serious illness. I shall do this by examining the issues of research, policy, and community and service development in the context of creating a broader health promoting environment for those who live with life-threatening or terminal illnesses.

The social experience that lies at the centre of most of the literature discussing support is obviously the 'support group' and particularly the 'self-help' group. The self-help group has been around for a long time. Claire Parkinson (1979), the author of what is still one of the best little primers on self-help groups available, argues that self-help groups can be observed in hunter-gatherer societies in the phenomena of food-gathering or safety groups. In the Middle Ages, self-help groups were the basis of medieval committees and guilds, while during the Industrial Revolution, self-help groups were also the basis of mutual-aid groups and were the forerunners of friendly societies (Parkinson 1979, pp. 2–3).

There is some debate about the meaning of the support group and its various categories, such as the self-help group. In this chapter I will review some of the main definitions of the support group, and I will review the strengths and weaknesses of this model of care. I will then provide a discussion of the relationship between health promotion and support groups before giving an overview of the use of support groups in cancer care. The practical issues concerning structure (organisation issues) and culture (social conduct issues) will then be discussed. Some practical 'rules' for the operation of the groups are suggested in that section.

DEFINITIONS

There is a lot of unnecessary complexity surrounding the idea of a 'support group'. Like the definition of health promotion itself, the basic idea behind the support group is quite simple. A support group is any collection of people who have similar needs that need addressing but that are not being addressed satisfactorily by others. Usually the support group is a small group—say, eight, ten, or fifteen people—who come together for the purposes of providing mutual aid, addressing common need, and facilitating personal and social exchange. Support groups are designed to support their members by meeting their needs.

Parkinson (1979, p. 7) describes two kinds of support groups: the 'redefiners' and the 'ameliorators'. The redefiners reject society's definition of them and seek to change it (for example, Black people, women, gay people, migrants, and so on). Ameliorators also reject society's definition of them, but they acknowledge that there is a problem inherent in their members' conditions (for example, members of Alcoholics Anonymous or Gamblers Anonymous). The best definition, however, is provided by the Council for the Single Mother and her Child (CSMC) (in Thorman 1987) and describes support groups as consisting of people with common attributes who get together to promote common interests.

Definitions such as the CSMC's have been criticised for being too broad and academically imprecise. Under this definition, service organisations, community groups, education programs, and even political groups can be included. We need not be too anxious about this lack of precision. We are not developing a social theory of support groups but merely attempting to convey what *most* of them are like in general, and what most of them are like in palliative care. And most of them are small groups of people with similar illness conditions who come together to help solve some common problems while providing each other with a measure of personal support. Some last for a few weeks, and others last for years. It is true that this definition might include some community groups or educational programs, but if this happens, we can speak of such groups as having support-group functions rather than being set up primarily for that purpose.

The other contentious issue that is raised by definitions of support groups is the issue of *who* leads them. Thomas Powell (1990) differentiates between 'autonomous' and 'hybrid' support groups. Autonomous support groups are led by people with the condition that causes them to come together—for example, cancer support groups are led by people with cancer. Hybrid support groups are led by professionals. If only life were as simple as some classification schemes seem to suggest! Many support groups are led by those who have had, but no longer have, the condition that 'causes the group to come together'. Other groups are indeed led by professionals, but these professionals may not be health professionals or are professionals who themselves have the condition that causes the group to come together.

Who leads the group is not very important. There are advantages and disadvantages either way. Obviously it is useful to have someone lead the group who has intimate knowledge and experience of the condition that brings the group together. But sometimes it can be useful to have an outsider to whom the group must verbalise their experiences so that they can clearly articulate their experiences to others. This can have additional advantages. As is the case in anthropological fieldwork, there are experiences and meanings that outsiders glean but that insiders regularly miss and vice versa.

Finally, not all professionals who run groups need to be 'professionals' from the health area, but may be chosen, or may choose to run support groups, because they bring particular experiences from their training in listening and facilitating. This can be useful. The problem with a person with the same condition leading the group may be similar to the problem that arises when someone takes a photograph of a group of friends: the friend taking the photo is left out.

STRENGTHS AND WEAKNESSES OF SUPPORT GROUPS

Parkinson (1979, pp. 14–17) provides an excellent summary of the advantages and disadvantages of support groups, and we shall review these here to establish their relevance, or otherwise, to health promoting palliative care.

In general, support groups may provide many functions that are consistent with a health promotion model of health care based on the Ottawa Charter. Support groups can be non-hierarchical and highly participatory. Groups without professional leadership are free of the professional relationships that emphasise the political, knowledge, or status differences between professionals and those who are not. If groups are led by professionals, and if these professionals view their role in primarily facilitative terms, such inequalities will seldom dominate the support groups' interactions.

Support groups also provide caring environments and assign humane and helping roles to all participants. Rather than receiving personal support from one source, most of the group can act together to provide a caring response to individual difficulties. By sharing problems and experiences with others, support groups can educate all participants by normalising their experiences within the group itself. In this way, the loneliness of individual experience can be placed in a broader social and health context.

Support groups can also be very flexible and responsive, meeting, as they often do, weekly or fortnightly. In this way, participants are able to update each other on the progress of their conditions and other people's responses to them. Support groups can also be flexible in another way. Groups can meet at times and places that are convenient for their members. They can meet at each other's homes or in local venues that are convenient to where most members live. Times can be arranged to fit in with work and child-care hours.

The coming together of a group of people with the same condition can also lead to the identification and better use of community and state resources, particularly when such groups act as lobby groups for more of those resources. Groups may network and liaise with similar groups to get better deals on medication or certain professional services. They can specialise their networking for greater efficiency and effectiveness.

The use and growth of certain types of support groups also act as a de facto critique of existing service arrangements. The growth of these groups can highlight the weaknesses in the current service provision arrangements. Such criticism can be influential in prompting new policy or funding developments, and can therefore be an important element in the push for changing attitudes in professional, community, and government circles.

Ultimately, of course, one of the key benefits of support groups is that they shift control back to users. This is itself one of the key strategies of an empowering health promotion. If this sense of control is not effectively supported, members of support groups quickly lose their interest and attendance drops. In the end, the usefulness of a support group is measured in terms of how well it is attended. If participants do not feel that the group is functioning to provide them with a measure of control and support in their difficulties, interest will wane.

Support groups are also excellent forums for strengthening and promoting change and participation. People come together to share and solve problems. They encourage each other to respond to each other's problems and to identify themselves with the group rather than simply regarding themselves as individuals. This can strengthen resolve and empower many to act as advocates for the group when faced with bureaucratic or professional resistance to issues that are important to the group.

Finally, support groups can be very informal and inexpensive. Beyond the initial shyness that people may experience on meeting strangers, support groups can provide low-key, low-threat means of support. For many people, the initial discomfort of meeting new people is quickly offset by the realisation of how much they have in common with their newly met support-group comrades.

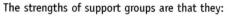

The strengths of support groups are that they:
- are non-hierarchical and participatory
- provide a caring environment
- are flexible and responsive
- facilitate specialised networking
- highlight weaknesses in current service provision
- shift control back to users
- strengthen and promote change
- are informal and inexpensive

Adapted from Parkinson 1979

There is little doubt that support groups can be important in the creation of supportive environments, and this is a key aim of the Ottawa Charter for Health Promotion. Furthermore, support groups have the potential to help participants to strengthen community action and develop personal skills. More informally, they may encourage a reorientation of both public policy and/or health services. In fact, their presence or existence alone can be regarded as a de facto reorientation of health services. The social and participatory nature of support groups makes them excellent vehicles for education, information, and interpersonal reorientation. In these ways, support groups are well suited to health promoting palliative care.

But it is not all good news. There are problems with, and criticism of, these types of groups, with some suggesting that support groups can work against an empowering style of health promotion. First, because many support groups are not based in institutions, there is a tendency for some of these to be non-accountable. The general impression of members that the group is meeting their aims may be based entirely on subjective impressions and tangible benefits in terms of actual learning. Objective improvement may, in fact, be minor or non-existent. Some groups may also be less than participatory in their decision-making, or allow certain ideas or people to dominate at the expense of others. There may be little provision for changing this situation other than splintering off into yet another support group.

Because groups begin informally, and are often led by those in similar situations, there can be a tendency within such a group to drift, creating ambiguity about the group's purpose and task. Issues to do with leadership and 'rules' about the conduct of the group can be the subject of tensions and conflict. In response to these problems, the group can become professionalised or bureaucratised, leading to rigidity of purpose and of process. This can further lead to a move away from the original participatory goals and philosophy of the support group.

Furthermore, if support groups grow in number and political strength, then rather than highlighting weaknesses in service provision, that growth may be used by some observers to argue that service provision is well in place. The success of support-group networks may actually lead to greater government apathy. Exacerbating this problem is the similar situation in which a 'ghetto' effect is produced by using only a very narrow range of services. By specialising, some support groups may not be encouraging better use of broader services and networks that may be of benefit to members. In this way, such specialised emphasis on a particular condition or problem may not encourage change in broad-er service systems. Specialisation can also lead to 'ghetto-isation' of a problem and of the groups who share this problem. Support groups can inadvertently legitimate and reinforce processes of marginalisation and inequality. Rather than encourage change, the growth of some support groups can entrench a resistance to change. It can also lead to easier identification of groups that are disliked or feared by prejudiced ele-ments of the community.

Finally, support groups can approach their problems, conditions, or experiences with the same, sometimes unhelpful, definitions of their situations as those held by professionals. Rather than providing an alternative view of their situation, some support groups can reinforce professional values and attitudes, which may be part of their difficulties. A 'fresh' examination of their experiences may be difficult to obtain, even away from ordinary professional encounters.

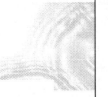

The weaknesses of support groups are that they:
- provide little accountability or program evaluation
- allow governments to maintain their apathy
- may attempt to overcome ambiguity by bureaucratising or professionalising
- do not encourage better use of broader networks
- can create the false impression that needs are being met
- legitimate marginalisation and inequality
- use the same problematic definitions as professionals

Adapted from Parkinson 1979

Let me address each one of these criticisms in their turn. First of all, the lack of accountability is not confined to informal support groups. Let us not forget that one of the key reasons for the rise of support groups is the lack of accountability and response on the part of con-ventional service providers. The issue of program evaluation is a mixed one. To the extent that members are *feeling* that their needs are being met, then that support group *is* actually doing the job well. The issue of objective or less impressionistic program evaluation is more about being accountable to others outside the group. If you are required to be accountable to funding bodies, for example, or to other people who feel that your 'say so' is not sufficient evidence, some kind of evaluation beyond impression will be valuable or even necessary. The purpose of the support group, and the desirability of stronger evidence of its value to members, is something that each group might decide about in its initial meetings. In the context of a health promoting palliative care, where such care is tied to other services, a careful program evaluation is crucial in accounting for the resources directed to these activities. It is also crucial in convincing others who are not an integral part of the service that such groups do indeed offer positive outcomes that are beyond reasonable dispute. Program evaluation is not optional in such contexts.

The problem of legitimating marginalisation or inequality for those living with dying would be a risk if all health promoting care were only about support groups. But it is *not* only about support groups. The curriculum, research, policy development, and service-reorientation functions of a health promoting palliative care are important counter-movements and strategies to prevent such marginalisation. They are also a defence against allowing governments to feel that appropriate services are already in place. Health promoting palliative care services, because they are not simply the provision of support groups, should also be active in reorienting both palliative care and public health services towards providing health promotion resources for those living with life-threatening or terminal illnesses. The linking of health promotion ideas with palliative care ideas, resource issues, and policy, curriculum, and research development is a move away from specialisation. This strat-egy ensures that health promoting palliative care is 'mainstreamed'— not with acute care or one of the other models of managed care that are so prevalent today, but with public health and its philosophy and policy mission.

As for the problems of professionalising and bureaucratising within the support groups themselves, some simple precautions can be put in place to safeguard against these tendencies. Groups should never be large; they should be confined to fifteen people or less. All participants should decide upon and agree to a basic list of 'rules' (or expectations). These should cover issues such as timing and venue, but also conventions about the purpose and style of the group. There should be general agreement on and legitimation of the values of listening, tolerance, and participation. We will return to this issue in the final section of this chapter.

SUPPORT GROUPS AND HEALTH PROMOTION

So, on balance, support groups are participatory group structures that are a flexible, responsive, and informal means of returning some measure of control to people whose problems are not adequately addressed by existing service-system provisions. But support groups are also valuable and excellent ways to achieve other goals in health promotion. For one thing, such groups provide encouragement, task reinforcement, and support for learning. They are themselves an important and highly effective context for learning.

Aside from providing simply caring environments, support groups are also able to provide a true and genuine empathy for their participants. As one self-helper put it: 'We share a greater depth of understanding—friends don't really understand—until you've walked the path you don't understand . . . I couldn't talk to my husband about some things but I could talk to a group member' (as quoted in Thorman 1987, p. 71)

And finally, self-help support groups can be started and maintained by anyone. Professional endorsement and involvement are not only unnecessary but also often undesired. In this way, support groups are a do-it-yourself (DIY) innovation and option in the health care area that have become increasingly popular because of their client-driven energy and purpose.

In these ways, the existence of support groups addresses four of the five principles of the Ottawa Charter for Health Promotion by:

- creating supportive environments
- strengthening community action
- developing personal skills
- bringing about the de facto reorientation of health services

Some observers have argued that support groups are largely middle-class phenomena and that they attract mainly women. This has been viewed as a criticism of support groups in general and implies that this strategy is less useful to other groups in society. There are several replies to this criticism and all of them are relevant to our discussion of health promoting palliative care. First, everyone dies. The fact that support groups have served mainly middle-class people and women is not a bad thing. Middle-class people and women deserve support services too. But it is not true that support groups serve *only* these groups. There is plenty of empirical evidence to suggest that members of other social classes and gender and ethnic groups are using support groups (see especially Thorman 1987). Second, the current pattern of support-group use may be less a function of preferences than it is the result of professional referral patterns. Several respondents comment about this in Thorman's (1987, pp. 60–1) research into Western Australian support groups:

(1) It is not easy to find [that] self help exists

(2) (apart from social workers) from other professionals . . . with rare exceptions there appears to be little referral

(3) It's hard to get doctors to tell their patients about the group . . . unless the person presents to him as being distressed, he doesn't tell them about the group

In general, and in Australia in particular, there may indeed be several factors influencing the use of support groups by the general community. There is often low general awareness about what support groups are able to achieve for their members, little public knowledge of the availability of such groups, and a lack of support for these groups from many of the professionals who refer clients. These factors contribute to less than optimal use of this form of health promotion. However, none of these factors has been adequately examined in the rush to critique the support group for underrepresentation—although these factors are clearly implicated. More research may help us to develop a more sober and scholarly evaluation of the extent of these problems.

Finally, one may argue that the support group is of little use in dealing with the problem and experience of end-stage dying. There are three points to make in connection with this criticism. First, we must remember that dying is not necessarily associated with slow deterioration. Many people die suddenly, and so the idea of 'end stage' must be critically checked against this counter-intuitive experience. Second, it is true that social support groups are best able to serve those who enjoy a reasonable level of health and who are ambulant. Nevertheless, this underscores the crucial importance of early referral. The best health and death education, and the longest lasting support (from any source), will always be initiated earlier rather than later. This is the ideal case scenario. For people who are encountered late in the course of their illness—who are besieged with tiredness or other difficult symptoms—support groups may be neither relevant nor desired. This observation notwithstanding, there are many who, late in the course of their illnesses, remain mentally alert and interested in their own and others' social and personal issues. Given a choice, these people may elect to join informal groups that meet casually and can provide important and satisfying sources of support and encouragement that they may not get otherwise. The important point is not to make the decision on behalf of clients or to withhold from them the opportunity for consultation that is given to those whose health may be better.

SUPPORT GROUPS IN PALLIATIVE CARE

The use of support groups in cancer care has been common in recent years and dates back to at least the early 1970s (Fobair 1997).They have also been commonly used in the HIV/AIDS area. The Long Island Association for AIDS Care, for example, has produced a very useful book on the structure and function of support groups for people living with AIDS (Barouh 1992). In the palliative care and psycho-oncology area, European and North American workers in the field have recently described the use and value of support groups. In Germany (Weiss et al. 1996), for example, the Tumour Biology Centre provides several types of support groups, which are used to provide music, art, occupational, and cognitive-behavioural therapies. The support groups in this program have a decidedly psychological and professional-led set of functions.The Canadian Hope and Cope program (Edgar et al. 1996) focuses much more on a social model of support group, using self-help groups to direct members' own education in areas of health, cosmetic information, and oncological information.This education occurs in a broader context of work with volunteers, and with library and public education services. The Hope and Cope program comes closest to resembling the health promotion ideals of a health promoting palliative care model.

It is not unusual for support groups to occur in the context of other support structures or programs, and the Canadian program is a good example of this in relation to cancer care. In the HIV/AIDS area, Gail Barouh (1992) describes how support groups can emerge from the individual self-identification of needs following a more structured and rather didactic forum. In this forum, four workshops are conducted to lead participants through information about the disease and various treatment options, survival strategies, legal and insurance issues, and issues related to intimacy, sex practices, and relationships in general.

There is a huge diversity of support groups, and of academic studies and evaluations of their effectiveness (see, for example, Iacovino & Reesor 1997; Fobair 1997). Some of these groups emphasise individual change; some emphasise information and learning; others are more problem-solving or outright therapeutic in nature, such as psychodrama groups (Nichols & Jenkinson 1991). Both Patricia Fobair (1997) and Keith Nichols and John Jenkinson (1991) argue that an eclectic approach is common, and most types of support group have reasonable evidence for their effectiveness. Vivian Iacovino and Kenneth Reesor (1997) observe that, despite some methodological reservations and criticism, most of the evaluation literature on psychosocial interventions, such as support groups, does suggest a positive impact on people's ability to adjust, especially to living with cancer.

So what are the 'positive impacts'? Yalom (1975) and Nichols and Jenkinson (1991) suggest that support groups in particular function to provide a sense of belonging. They can also provide a sense of universality of feeling, of 'normalness' about one's responses to a certain experience or knowledge. Support groups provide people with hope, honest feedback, and vicarious learning opportunities through listening and watching others. Finally, support groups provide people with a safe site to express feelings and thoughts, as well as the support for personal change if this is desired. Intellectual growth through structured learning and the gathering of new information is also one of the important benefits of participating in support groups.

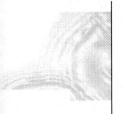

The positive impacts of support groups are that they:
- provide a sense of belonging
- normalise experience and response
- provide hope, honest feedback, and vicarious learning
- are a safe site for feelings, thoughts, and change
- facilitate learning and information gathering

Edgar and colleagues (1996) in their review of the evaluation literature on support groups found that there tended to be an improvement in participants' general health perception, and of their body image and the management of feelings. Other studies reported a decrease in tension and in depression, particularly in older cancer patients (Hann et al. 1995). Other evaluations have reported increases in self-reported quality of life and the amelioration of psychosocial problems. More controversial have been the reports of increased survival rates compared with those who have not participated in such groups (Fawzy et al. 1995).

It seems from the above review that:

1 support groups are generally beneficial, and are certainly often perceived as such by both participants and a methodologically broad and diverse evaluation literature
2 groups that facilitate personal support and expressivity may be marginally better for participants (Fobair 1997, p. 77)
3 they are effective both in the context of professional supervision and without such supervision, and with or without other supports, such as libraries or structured supplementary education programs

They are suitable, then, for broad health promoting programs of various types—either DIY, out-patient, in-patient, or as part of an outreach pastoral care service.

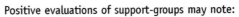

Positive evaluations of support-groups may note:
- improvement of general health perception
- improvement of body image and management of feelings
- reduction in tension and depression
- increase in vigour and self-reported quality of life
- increase in survival rates

From a health promoting palliative care viewpoint, we need to factor in the broad concerns of health and death education, and of interpersonal reorientation, as the primary—but not necessarily sole—concerns of any support group. These concerns can be addressed to greater or lesser degrees by individual groups, depending on their particular needs and decisions.

Clearly, though, a health promoting support group is not one that provides an essentially therapeutic, psychological response to living with dying. I have discussed this earlier in the chapter on health education. The primary responsibility of support groups is to access information and to help those living with serious illness to solve social, health-related, and death-related problems. In this sense, then, health promoting palliative care support groups are basically self-help groups in terms of their broad purpose.

SOME PRACTICAL ISSUES

If you have never before run a support group, there are several practical issues that you will need to consider. A good support group is also a good learning environment, and so if you have ever run a university tutorial group, discussion seminar, or community reading group, then you might draw on some of these experiences.

Good organisation and a supportive culture are essential ingredients for a successfully run support group. You will need to consider size. Larger groups can be more difficult because they do not provide easy opportunities for everyone to speak. Larger groups can also be daunting for participants, and some people use the size of a group to 'hide' themselves. Groups that contain between ten and fifteen people are optimum. Anything larger and it becomes more difficult for everyone to participate fully and actively. On the other hand, small groups with only three or four members can be very intense and can lead to heightened self-consciousness on the part of some individuals. Also, it is easier to see some people's views as functions of their personalities rather than the result of broader social experience when there are no other individuals in the group who display a similar attitude or who identify with a similar type of experience. This inability to easily sort psycho-logical from social experiences can be unhelpful.

After the initial venue for the first meeting has been decided, meet-ing times and the frequency of meetings need also to be worked out, and this might occur in consultation with group members at that ini-tial meeting. At this time too, the duration of the meetings needs to be discussed. I find 2 hours to be just the right amount of time, with some groups finishing earlier if there is a sense within the group that it should finish earlier on a particular day. Nichols and Jenkinson (1991), who have written extensively on these practical issues (and have pro-duced a work worth consulting), recommend that meetings last between 1 hour and 1½ hours.

You will also need to decide about the group's aims. The most important issue here will be to decide how much time should or could be devoted to expressive support in relation to time spent in active learning tasks. The composition of the group also needs some thought. Will people with HIV/AIDS join the same group as people with can-cer? Will men and women belong to the same group (or, to put this in different terms, will women whose primary illness is cancer of the breast belong to the same groups as men with prostate cancer)? What are the implications of separating these people, and of keeping them together? These questions highlight the broader problem of inclusion criteria.

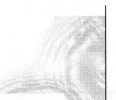

Organisational issues for support groups:
- size of the group
- venue
- meeting frequency and times
- duration of meetings
- aims of the group
- composition of the group (inclusion criteria)

Nichols and Jenkinson (1991, pp. 68–80) suggest that it is useful to think about the following issues:

- participants' willingness to listen
- confidentiality
- the relationship between dominating and shy personalities
- the importance of looking for answers rather than supplying them
- psychiatric or behavioural problems
- participants' acceptance of the broad ideals of health promotion

Clearly, support groups can manage people who are shy or dominating, but you will need to work out careful and sensitive strategies for dealing with these kinds of people should you decide on their inclusion. Also, support groups work well for people with behavioural or psychiatric problems, but usually in support groups specifically for those kinds of problems. In other support groups, for other purposes, the risk of serious disruption needs to be considered carefully. It is important to obtain participants' acceptance of the broad ideals of support groups in health promotion if the group is not to be at cross-purposes with these ideals. Barouh (1992) suggests a set of 'rules' (or 'guiding principles' or 'expectations') that might be read by a group and signed by them before joining a support group. Another way to bring these ideals to the attention of group members is to list them on a wall poster. The palliative care unit where I work takes this approach. I reproduce that poster here, not as a set of rules to follow, but as an example that you may use in developing your own thoughts about what 'rules' may be relevant to the conditions and needs of your own support group.

Did you know?
- The group is for *you* and you alone.
- Groups are *all* their members—attendance *is* important.
- Groups start on time.

- If you are late or unable to attend, we are grateful for a phone call from you.
- This is a drug-free space (including tobacco and alcohol).
- Everything we discuss in this room is confidential.
- Everyone is entitled to be heard.
- Tolerance is our way, not criticism.
- *Your* answers may not be someone else's.
- Erroneous information will be corrected by facilitators.

Courtesy of the Palliative Care Unit, La Trobe University

Finally, but just as importantly, do not be demoralised when some groups simply 'don't work'. Every year I lead dozens of groups, and every year there is one group that, no matter what I try, simply seems unable to talk with each other or is dominated by one or two people, despite my best efforts. Be patient. Learn from experience. Persevere.

6

Interpersonal Reorientation

The problem of community,

which is the form of personal life,

is the one of deciding on whose terms

it shall be lived.

Robert O. Johann, as quoted in

Savary et al. 1970, p. 211

Most of our clinical understanding of dying comes from institutional sources (hospitals, hospices) which focus on the last few weeks or days of dying. However, the prospect of death promotes personal and social changes that begin with the initial awareness that a current illness is life-threatening. Such an experience or event can continually alter the behaviour and attitudes of the individual and others, reorienting the identity of the self through changed interaction between the individual and significant others.

Given the numerous changing circumstances and responses experienced by individuals, we should note at the outset of this chapter that there is no such entity as 'the dying person'. In other words, although we can compile a sociological and historical 'identikit' picture of dying in terms of idealised and typical conduct and experiences, this picture will rarely, if ever, 'fit' any one particular individual. Similarly, social pictures of 'the migrant experience', 'the working-class experience', or 'the student radical' type, for example, will provide a set of characteristics that can sensitise us to *possible* features that we may encounter in real individuals who have undergone some type of experience or share some common types of values. But the composite social pictures can never *be* the real, personal examples. If we try to see people in these ways, we can be rightly accused of stereotyping them. In this chapter we aim to sensitise ourselves to the possible circumstances and social influences that help to shape people's personal and social experiences. In this way, we are able to see the *range* of possibilities to which people with life-threatening or terminal illnesses are subject.

People are beings at the centre of a web of human relationships, financial commitments, and institutional obligations. They tend, in that context, to resist major changes in their lives unless the forces are considerable. The social and personal impact of serious illness can be significant. Few people, in the event of serious illness, experience no change at all. The reorientation of self that must accompany such changes is only appreciated when one acknowledges the number and diversity of changes to which the dying person must adjust. This chapter, therefore, provides a basic, but not exhaustive, review of those changes, many of which will be part of the daily exchanges in support groups and one-on-one discussions. We will begin by considering a person's 'usual life', identify some of the major changes of circumstances that can occur, and then discuss the range of possible responses to those changes. The review will cover emotional life, family life, work life, sex and recreational life, spiritual life, and health care experiences.

EMOTIONAL LIFE

It is often true that people cope with the stress of bad news in the same ways that they have coped with negative experiences in the past. These familiar ways of coping might be viewed as benchmarks of coping for all of us. However, a poor prognosis can prompt a number of possible fears that may not be within the scope of past experiences and their habitual reactions. Foremost among such fears must be the prospects of death, disfigurement, dependency, and radically altered personal futures. These can be significant sources of anxiety, anger, or depression. In the HIV/AIDS area, for example, C. G. Lyketsos and colleagues (1996), and Judd and colleagues (1997) report significantly higher rates of psychiatric morbidity among people with HIV/AIDS than in the general population or in other medical out-patient medical clinics. Such fears can also lead to a grieving process that can go unnoticed if one is not sensitised to these specific personal sources. At the very least, a period of introversion or meditation on these worries might be expected in some people.

These four concerns—death, disfigurement, dependency, and loss of personal futures—are regularly reported in the literature on psychosocial needs of people with cancer (Bunston et al. 1995; Charles et al. 1996; Roberts et al. 1997) and AIDS (Schofferman 1988).

Emotional Life

Changed circumstances	– prospect of death
	– disfigurement
	– dependency
	– loss of future
Possible responses	– *anxiety or depression*
	– *loss and grief*
	– *introversion*

Death means different things to different people, but among the core concerns might be fear of abandonment, fear of simply not existing, or fear of some form of religious judgment. The prospect of leaving friends or relatives forever can also create a terrible sense of anguish and loss. The fear of a recurrence of the disease can be anchored in, or be a mask for, these kinds of fears.

The fear of disfigurement can also haunt many people. Individuals who are confronting a cancer of the neck, throat, or head may hold legitimate concerns in this area. Women with breast cancer commonly hold this fear also, fearing the loss of a breast or its disfigurement through 'lumpectomy'. Some men may harbour similar (but unfounded) fears over prostate cancer, while more generally, people may fear hair loss through chemotherapy or radiotherapy.

Aside from death and disfigurement, people may also fear dependency. Although this is a key fear of older people in general, it is also a key fear for young people (Roberts et al. 1997) and people with HIV/AIDS (Schofferman 1988). One suspects that this is a fear that most of us would share, irrespective of age or disease state. The fear of abandonment that grows from a sense of vulnerability can create ambivalence or tension when such a fear coexists with a fear of dependency.

Furthermore, Terry Bunston and others (1995) argue that a strong internal locus of control is a key determinant in maintaining hope. The idea that one still controls one's own life, and that personal outcomes are still significantly influenced by one's own decision-making and actions, is important. A sense of dependency can undermine or challenge that internal sense of control and can have negative consequences for a person's usual emotional responses to a health crisis, such as the diagnosis of a life-threatening illness.

Finally, news of a poor prognosis can generate a fear or set of concerns revolving around the idea of a lost future. Young adults with cancer, for example, can grieve over the loss of a career, or the prospect of not having a family or marriage partner. But older people can also experience this sense of loss, with some people looking forward to a long retirement in order to fulfil dreams that they could not realise in a full and busy work life. It goes without saying that the occurrence of cancer in mid-career, or while family are not quite grown up, has a similar impact and causes similar concerns.

FAMILY LIFE

The usual family life of most individuals revolves around a routine of daily activities that may have, at their core, paid employment, daily chores, or patterns of activity that relate to major hobbies or work-seeking activities. In that context, the pattern of social visits by others, and a person's interactions with others at home, will be underpinned by taken-for-granted assumptions about conduct. For instance, a certain friend might always call around once every three weeks, or a certain family member might always do the cooking or take the kids to and from school every day. Illness, or the simple public announcement of a life-threatening illness, can change any of these patterns and routines.

On the negative side, routines may be altered by poor health. Illness and treatment may impose new physical limits. But the kindness of others and the generous willingness of others to be of service may also alter a person's taken-for-granted routines. On the other hand, the news of seroconversion or a diagnosis of cancer may lead to social rejection, not only by distant friends and associates, but also by close friends or even spouses. Positive HIV status or a cancer that affects the cervix or breast may generate fears of contamination or disfigurement in *others*, and this, on rare occasions, has led to spouses deserting their partners (Leviton 1978). More often, the news of a life-threatening illness will only contribute negatively if the existing relationship has already been deteriorating (Kellehear 1990, p. 92).

Such experiences highlight the general problem of inequality in relationships with people with life-threatening or terminal illnesses (Kellehear 1994). Experiences of inequality may be frank, open, and underpinned by rejection and discrimination, but at least as many of these experiences may come from well-meaning people whose intent is entirely positive and altruistic. Out of a desire to 'help' or 'support' their spouse or friend, many people too quickly cast those friends in a 'sick role'. In that way, a person's usual roles, routines, or activities may be taken away from them without negotiation or their request. For fear of appearing ungrateful or unappreciative, many of those people with life-threatening illnesses will not object or protest. People too quickly make the judgment that others who are in personal trouble are personally inadequate. It may not be the case. People with chronic illnesses have their 'good days' and their 'bad days', and many of their associates are remiss in not consulting with their sick friends about that cycle of experience and adjusting their well-meaning behaviour accordingly. Unless they do so, undesirable role reversals and feelings of inequality and resentment can occur in the 'helped' one.

Family life	
Changed circumstances	– altered routines
	– rejection
	– inequality
	– increased closeness

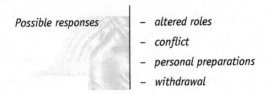

Possible responses
- altered roles
- conflict
- personal preparations
- withdrawal

There may also be positive changes to a person's family life. Some people may experience greater closeness to a partner or the family as a whole. Crises can sometimes draw families and friends together in ways that are rewarding to the person with illness. An increase in the number of visitors and new friends made in treatment centres can be experienced as a positive development in a person's life, sometimes reducing the sense of isolation that the person may have experienced before the illness. The new friends and added attention can be perceived as supportive and welcome.

The prospect of death can also tempt people to initiate a series of actions within their families that they may not have ordinarily engaged in without such a threat. For example, many older women may engage in 'informal willing' (Kellehear 1990). Women whose lives were mainly spent in domestic, rather than paid, employment activities may see some of their preparations for death in terms of seeing that certain private and valued items 'go' to their children before their deaths. This is a variation on the conduct often displayed by older couples who desire to see their children enjoy their gifts while they are still alive and well rather than to bequeath those goods and chattels later. Other people wish to open discussions with their partners about remarrying. Some people with terminal illnesses wish to assist in clarifying these issues with their partners so that their partners do not feel a sense of guilt or betrayal after the death of their current spouse. Any of the above changes to family life brought about by illness, treatment, or the knowledge of prognosis can lead to increased conflict, or an alteration to the usual patterns of conflict in a family.

One unrecognised additional source of conflict is often the occurrence of a near-death experience. Either during a treatment routine or during a particularly critical time in an episode of illness, a person may experience a near-death experience. Although the psychological features of the experience are well known (out-of-body sensations, life review, tunnel sensations, meetings with white lights or deceased relatives), less recognised are the changes to character and personal values that may occur in the wake of such experiences. Dissatisfaction with other values, assumptions, or attitudes—formerly one's own—in one's spouse, work, or family life can precipitate or increase family conflict. For the people who must relate to this 'new' character or set of personal changes, this can be a tense and perplexing time. They may be mystified as to why the person they thought they knew could be so changed by the simple occurrence of a 'passing hallucination' during an illness or treatment episode. It is not just the facts of illness, treatment, or prognosis, but also incidents such as a resuscitation event, that can create complications and changes in the family life of those at the centre of such experiences. Near-death experiences are powerful mechanisms for personal reorientation, which can be equally powerful in disorienting a person's family and usual supports.

WORK LIFE

As with family life, few workplaces are unchanged or unmoved by the news, if they receive it, of a colleague experiencing serious illness. The workplace is usually the cosy home of office politics, with a person's place in that game dependent on both personality and position. However, few people are so caught up in that web of chessboard concerns that they are unable to understand the deeper human issues raised by an illness such as metastatic cancer or AIDS. That insight alone is enough to embolden employers and employees to act, mostly in a positive way.

It is true that openly discriminatory practices might occur, such as dismissal, but there are currently laws in most places that make such an act a less than desirable employer response to anyone with cancer or AIDS. Nevertheless, dismissal may occur. Just as seriously, problems in the workplace may be more covert and insidious. Being 'passed over' for promotion, receiving less support for staff development and training, receiving less encouragement to attend public engagements, and other missed opportunities may be motivated by either rejecting or supportive attitudes. It is not always easy to tell, even when one is provided with an ostensibly positive explanation. Work friends may be less enthusiastic about inviting one to after-work functions, particularly social functions, for fear of contagion or because the seriously ill person may symbolically have a dampening effect on a gathering. This has been called the experience of stigma—the problem of 'spoiled identity' (Goffman 1974).

It is more likely, however, that workplaces will be sites of popularity for the seriously ill person (Kellehear 1990). Colleagues can provide assistance with the person's usual duties. Employers may request such assistance on behalf of the ill employee. Breaks may be provided so that the person who is ill can attend medical appointments, or observe a particular dietary or meditation regime. None of this might have been requested. The employer may transfer the employee who is ill to lighter duties or arrange extra 'sick day' provisions. Work colleagues have been known to 'pass the hat' around to supply extra money for treatments, for special holiday treats, or to pay for airfares to sacred religious sites such as Lourdes or Fatima. There is no telling in what special way a circle of supportive work friends may act. Anything is possible, and many of these possibilities have been documented in personal narratives of cancer or HIV illness in the workplace.

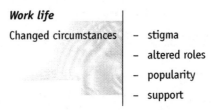

Work life

Changed circumstances

- stigma
- altered roles
- popularity
- support

	– declining work performance
	– over-protection
	– sacking
	– discrimination
	– gossip
	– funds generation
Possible responses	– *additional workplace stresses*
	– *financial and/or legal preparations*

But whether workplace reaction is positive or negative, in certain instances or in general, those alterations invariably bring with them a higher level of perceived stress. Attention, desirable or otherwise, is usually unsuspected and novel, and requires a certain degree of reorientation and adjustment. There is no accounting for what people will do, and when one steps outside the usual routines of work, people can come up with the unexpected regularly.

Aside from the events and actions taken by others in the workplace that may require a certain degree of social reorientation, the prospect of death may also encourage the person with a life-threatening illness to initiate his or her own agenda. Most often these actions concern overt preparations for death that relate in some way to income and financial security, particularly for families. At other times, financial hardship can be a concern for many who find themselves chronically ill and confronting mounting bills—medical or otherwise (Schulz et al. 1995). The issues that seem to be important are those that relate to superannuation, funeral costs, funding for treatments and medications, additional transport costs, or the creation of special bank accounts to help survivors cope with a person's death and subsequent loss of income. Several writers comment on the dominance of these concerns when living with a serious and potentially life-threatening illness (see Charles et al. 1996 and Roberts et al. 1997).

At some time, a person with serious illness may visit bankers, lawyers, accountants, and funeral businesses, in an effort to place his or her 'affairs in order'. This conduct may be new to both the dying person and his or her peers and family, and might be of concern to both. What is 'realistic' behaviour for one person may be interpreted as 'giving up hope' or prematurely resigning oneself to death in others. At these times too, general practitioners may be asked questions about donation of organs or volunteering for experimental medical programs in an effort to 'be of use to someone—even when dying' (Kellehear 1990).

Not everyone who works, works in paid employment. There are significant numbers of women, for example, who work at home. Many of these people take pride in that work and may feel equally distressed about losing their usual roles and responsibilities. This is another area that is not well recognised, but such change in household work activities, if it occurs, can be significantly disorienting for the worker.

Finally, employers—those who are company owners or who are self-employed—may also initiate changes at the news of their own poor prognosis. Relief workers may need to be employed, or a changeover within business or family circles may need to be initiated. Selling the business may also need to be considered or actively planned for. These events may not have been organised or anticipated before news of the illness, and can be additional fuel to a sense of loss and grief.

SEX AND RECREATIONAL LIFE

Sex is a topic about which much nonsense has been written, and in respect to terminal illness, that tradition continues. The major problem is that most writers consistently refuse to recognise the *changing nature* of the course of illness, the idiosyncratic patterns of sexual need and habit within humanity, and the diverse way in which people can express sexual desire aside from sexual intercourse. There is little doubt that treatments can adversely affect sexual desire and/or performance. There is also little doubt that sexual activity is not foremost in the minds of people hours before their deaths. Nevertheless, aside from these extreme and difficult events, sexual desire and activity are a normal and usual part of living, and that includes living with dying.

Nevertheless, problems in the area of sexual activity are commonly reported by a minority of those who participate in studies of this area. Charles and others (1996) and Roberts and colleagues (1997) report that about 20 per cent of their respondents reported some difficulties in sexual activity as part of the life changes affecting people living with cancer. In a study of life changes affecting people living with terminal cancer, I reported that slightly more than half of the 69 sexually active respondents reported problems (Kellehear 1990). In most cases, each of the studies reported a generally decreasing level of sexual activity. For some people, sexual activity ceased with recurrence of the illness. Pain or discomfort were key reasons for decreasing or cessation of sexual activity. Sometimes anxiety or depression interfered with desire or motivation.

At other times, changes in physical appearance dampened motivation. Self-consciousness about altered body image because of surgery or other treatment interventions made some people disinclined to initiate. The physical symptoms of disease seem to be the main deterrent to sexual activity for most people experiencing problems. Sexual desire, on the other hand, often remained. There is no necessary association, therefore, between decreased activity and desire. In the light of this, there may be a need for information about norms in this area, as well as for strategies to overcome physical difficulties.

Sex and recreational life

Changed circumstances	– physical restrictions
	– altered needs
	– altered appearance
	– popularity
Possible responses	– *increased, decreased, or high-risk sexual activity*
	– *isolation*
	– *busyness*

There have been reports of hypersexuality as a result of terminal prognosis in cancer (Raphael & Maddison 1972) and HIV/AIDS, but this is an uncommon response. Nevertheless, hypersexuality is one of several responses to life-threatening illness that must be recognised as a possible area of social reorientation for those with life-threatening illnesses.

Safe-sex practices may also slip away under these comparatively new social conditions when safe sex is not the usual sexual practice of that individual. Among a small sample of HIV positive men, Brian Kelly and others (1991, p. 370) found that 'depression correlated positively with frequency of high-risk sexual practices'. Recognition of those risks, and attention to their rectification, should occur as early as possible—a point crucial in any health promotion program.

Recreational activities can be reduced because of increasing isolation, because of progressive illness and physical restriction, or through the social rejection and withdrawal of others. Cancer sufferers commonly report increased social popularity, characterised by a sharply increased number of social visits, family reunions, and phone calls. Many make new friends through this activity or among health care professionals and patients who they meet in frequenting health care institutions. But there are stories of rejection too. Some people do report losing contact with some friends and relatives because of ignorance, despair, or fear. Myths that AIDS or cancer are punishment for wrongdoing, or are as contagious as the common cold, are still believed by a few unfortunate people in every community.

Although we regularly read of people with a terminal illnesses going on spending sprees, visiting Europe, or buying red Porsches, a far more realistic picture is that of the chronically ill person in front of the television. This is a less glamorous and far less reported image of living with dying, but one that is closer to the mark. Because tiredness is so often a problem, listening to music, watching television, or reading are major activities. Simply lying for hours on one's back and thinking or day-dreaming can be an equally common activity.

Nevertheless, it must be noted that significant numbers of people report little change in their recreational lives. Some people take on passive recreational pursuits in addition to their active pastimes, and others substitute those active recreational pursuits for passive ones. No dominant pattern of response is easy to discern here. The important point to remember in connection with patterns of changed recreational life is that slow physical deterioration is not necessarily related to slow dying (Witzel 1975).

SPIRITUAL LIFE

In this section I am employing the term 'spiritual' as an umbrella term that includes not only religious beliefs, values, and activities, but also the more broadly existential issues. I include a concern about 'life beyond death' as a 'religious' concern because this is an essentially eschatological (or pareschatological) issue—an issue concerning thoughts about the final resting place and destiny of souls. By 'existential' I mean concerns about the ultimate meaning of things—life, death, purpose, work, relationships, hope, and so on.

Much of the shocking impact of life-threatening and terminal illnesses lies in the fact that their sufferers may die more quickly than they would ordinarily anticipate. In other words, this means that thoughts about death are entertained much earlier, for most people, than they would have desired. People tend to think that thoughts about personal death, as opposed to the death of others, will occur late in life. That, however, is not always the way it happens. The fact seems to be that few people in our society are encouraged to think about death or dying, and so death nearly always remains a shocking event.

Putting the sadness and loss associated with any death aside for one moment, one of the lingering problems that people are left to wrestle with is the problem of how to reorient to a radically different, often vague, and highly contentious 'future'. Within some people's belief systems, there is no personal survival of death. For these people, death is regarded as a final oblivion, annihilation. Meaning is to be sought, if it can be rescued at all, in some kind of reorganisation of feeling, memory, and reflection about their lives so far and their remaining time.

For other people, finding meaning with regard to their prospects is about rescuing the fragments of an earlier religious education and piecing those fragments together in new ways that they might now find meaningful. At least a third of the 100 respondents in my own study of people with terminal cancer responded in this way, returning to regular prayer, church attendance, or regular engagement with clergy (Kellehear 1990, p. 131). The reasons for this return to orthodoxy lay in their belief that these activities provided them with an important source of social support.

For a small group of people, though, the idea of an afterlife and the personal need to 'make peace' with God was an important concern. For those who have a pre-existing religious commitment that is not related to their recent illness, the idea of reunion—with deceased friends and God—can and does supply a measure of comfort and only requires minor personal reorientation.

Spiritual life	
Changed circumstances	– prospect of no future
	– reunion with those 'gone before'
	– prospect of meeting God
	– vague notions of 'afterlife'
Possible responses	– *return to religious observance*
	– *altered reading habits*
	– *the company of clerics*
	– *hedonistic responses*

In addition to the possibility of a return to religious observance and the need for the social support of clerics and others within religious communities, the prospect of death for a small group of people may elicit a hedonistic response. In those cases where the prospect of death means the permanent annihilation of personal consciousness and experience, a very few people may respond by spending all their money and/or engaging in thrill-seeking and otherwise high-risk behaviour that may endanger both themselves and others. Such a response may not always be as spectacular as these sentences may initially imply. Heavy or binge drug use, for example, can be one of the subtle ways that reckless feelings and thoughts can be expressed. High-risk drug use or sexual behaviour can be a response to materialist ideas about death, but these behaviours might be new, and therefore additionally disorienting for these people. A moderate drinker can suddenly become a binge or heavy drinker. A casual smoker of cannabis can become a heavy user, or expand that use into 'harder' drugs.

Other people may alter their reading habits, soaking up every book ever written on the meaning of life, the near-death experience, or spiritualism. The pursuit of existential and religious answers can become an obsession and can replace their usual recreational pursuits for a period. Peter's story (as quoted in Barouh 1992, pp. 7–8) is a good example. He describes his first reaction to the news of being HIV positive:

> I don't know how I reacted when I first found out. Basically, I did a lot of running around. In order not to become hysterical about the situation, I decided to try and take control, and I went out and bought everything I could read . . . that was probably my way of not dealing with the feelings that were going on. But it worked for me and it kept me on a fairly even keel for the first couple of months.

The desire to reorient to existential and religious possibilities, either as a way of mapping possible futures, or as a way to find some broader meaning in the current pattern of suffering and loss, can be important. Responding to this desire is a social reorientation and support function that death education can provide. The spiritual buttressing and support that can occur in that education is one of the broader aspects of 'health pro-motion' that derives from the palliative care discourse and assumptions.

HEALTH CARE EXPERIENCES

Although nearly everyone has at least one relationship with a health care provider, most of the time that relationship is occasional. Chronic illness brings people into the health care system on a regular basis and puts them into regular contact with many different providers. It does so through the provision of treatments, both 'active' and palliative.

For most people, the initial news about their disease is received in the context of a long-term trust in the authority of the health care provider, usually the specialist or general practitioner. However, the shock of the news and the enormity of its possible implications for lifestyle and life span can sometimes prompt people to seek another opinion. For some people this is like 'shopping around,' ensuring that they have the most accurate advice available, ensuring that there is little doubt about their illness. For others, it may be about buying some breathing space in order to accept the seriousness of the situation—a kind of graduated, self-controlled way of confronting the problem. For some other people, this seeking of second or third or fourth opinions represents a reluctance to face up to the life-threatening nature or pres-ence of the illness. In any case, underlying all these searches for clarifi-cation is the attempt, one way or another, to achieve some kind of reorientation towards one's new identity as someone with a chronic and serious illness.

Health care experiences	
Changed circumstances	– diverse and increased professional contacts
	– 'active' and palliative treatments

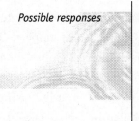

Possible responses	– *second or more opinions*
	– *complementary therapy*
	– *aggressive pursuit of experimental treatments*
	– *increased closeness and care for providers*

When medical opinion has been exhausted or accepted, some people try alternative forms of health care treatment. For some people, this is a complementary strategy designed to augment their medical treatments. Some people may substitute their medical treatments for complementary ones. Although only a small minority of people with terminal cancer seem to seek alternative therapists (Kellehear 1990, p. 109), a significant number of these are younger, educated people. This suggests that for illnesses such as AIDS, the minority may not be so small. Furthermore, as the educated 'baby-boomers' move into high cancer-risk age groups, more and more of these can be expected to explore alternative healing options.

Not all people will explore complementary therapy by visiting practising therapists such as aromatherapists, herbalists, acupuncturists, and so on. Some may simply read about 'cancer cures' in books and try the numerous diets recommended by this genre of literature. Other people will rely on advice from well-meaning friends and even their own memories of television programs seen years earlier. Such advice or memories may prompt them to take high doses of vitamin C or to begin hoarding almond or pumpkin kernels. Other people may draw on fable and begin, for example, to chew basil leaf regularly in the belief that, rather than being an antidote to a basilisk's fatal stare, it may stave off the spectre of death. I interviewed a man once who shyly confessed to chewing small amounts of 'wandering Jew' growing wild in his backyard in the private belief that this might cure him.

The task of health promotion in these contexts is to ensure maximum accuracy of information about complementary services, products, and ideologies, and to be able to balance an interest in these areas with sympathetic, but critical, information support. Other people are vulnerable to extreme religious or social groups who make out-rageous claims about the treatments they offer. We all know of people who would be more than willing to spend their life savings to fly to a foreign country or charismatic 'healer' to seek a cure that 'medicine denies'. The task of a participatory health promotion is to provide the best available information about these services and perhaps, within self-help groups, to explore the reasoning behind the desire for such treat-ments. At the end of the day, however, the decision rests with the participant. But because the complementary therapy world may be new and unfamiliar, reliable information will be crucial to orientation towards it.

Apart from those who become great fans of the alternative, there are a small number of people who become 'groupies' of orthodox medical treatment. If it is available, they want some of it—now. These are the people who believe that more treatments are better than none, or that the more aggressive the treatment, the better their prospects, or that if they are going to die anyway, they might as well volunteer as 'guinea pigs' for science. Once again, whatever the motivation, it is useful to explore some of the reasoning behind such approaches, as well as the risks and benefits. People do not always realise that a treatment can be worse for them than the illness.

Finally, it is common for some people with chronic illness in gener-al, and life-threatening illness in particular, to develop an increased interest in the health and welfare of their health care providers. Some people put the needs of their doctors (as they perceive them) before their own, wishing to 'spare' their practitioners from disappointment or additional stress (Kellehear & Fook 1989). Yet other people come to feel close to their doctors, and are keen to erode the professional distance between them and their providers during this stressful time for both. Issues of transference and counter-transference can be highlighted at these times and for these relationships (Vafiadis 1997). The closeness that may come about does not necessarily present a problem to patients or health care providers, and can be one of the more rewarding and positive aspects of health care for both. Many a genuine and beneficial friendship has been born from these kinds of developments, with many benefits, not the least being the enhancement of trust and support for both parties.

REORIENTING THE SELF

In this chapter I have provided a broad summary of the range of changes to which people living with serious illness must adapt and respond within the major social situations they encounter. I must emphasise that these changes are not the only ones that people encounter, but they are among the major changes reported by the research and clinical literature. It is difficult to say which of these changes do, or do not, apply to people in their last days or hours of life. This is because, as mentioned earlier, people do not always follow a path of slow deterioration. Sudden death is common, with many people being ambulant and reasonably well up to their last day on Earth. Others may follow a slow path of deterioration—what sociologists Barney Glaser and Anselm Strauss (1968) have described as a 'trajectory'. Even here, though, the problems encountered in the social interaction during the final hours of life may correspond to some of the difficulties discussed earlier—as well as others.

I was once told about a woman who was 'days from dying' in a hospice but who suddenly became very enthusiastic about a certain treatment for cancer that she had just read about in a well-known women's magazine. Some may entertain psychological theories about such enthusiasm so late in the course of her illness. In social terms, however, the hope that this woman displayed about her situation demanded support. Providing information about the treatment and its possible use to her at her stage of illness may restore or maintain her sense of control at this time, whether or not she is able to access the treatment itself. A sense of hope and control are good for morale, and this can be 'health promoting'.

But aside from individual cases, we are able to identify eight strategies for assisting and encouraging interpersonal reorientation to the changes that living with serious illness brings about for many people.

1 One can *provide information* on what is usual for those living with life-threatening or terminal illnesses. A photocopy of this chapter or the recommendation of any of the many good books available about living with chronic illness will be valuable here. Specific information about common sexual problems or fears and ways to overcome them will also be valuable. Issues to do with risk-taking conduct—whether sex-related or drug-related—might be addressed with some harm-reduction strategies and advice.

2 It is crucial that professional people *provide listening and discussion opportunities*, either in one-to-one situations or in support-group contexts. This is important for consciousness raising, and for the sharing and solving of problems. People need information, but sometimes that information is derived from listening to themselves reflect about their own situations. For others, listening carefully is about maximising the opportunity to understand their situation so that correct information and appropriate support are provided. This issue is related to the third point.

3 *Make time, and make it repeatedly.* Problems come and go. Not everyone is ready to discuss things that are causing concern all at once. Some people like to choose their time, their confidante, or their context. Others take time to muster courage or to feel comfortable. New problems emerge and old ones can return in new guises. Reorienting is continual because the disease keeps changing, as life itself does, right up to the last minute.

4 *Provide role-play opportunities* for those who may be helped by 'practising' stress-breaking strategies. Assertion training can be gained by 'acting' the conduct that people fear. Sometimes acting out the

problem with others can provide insights into behaviour that are not gained by simply describing the problem to others. Role plays may be useful strategies for some people.

5 It is important to *provide relevant reference material*. I have discussed some of this in chapter 4 (on death education), but the point is worth repeating. It can be useful to keep taped talks or books and articles on hand to lend to clients who may be interested in the social, physical, psychological, or spiritual questions relevant to their current situation. The use of guest speakers—doctors, lawyers, or accountants for example—should be included in this way.

6 *Information evenings for families, friends, and employers* will also be useful. Remember that only so much can be achieved by people with serious illness. These people exist in the context of relationships with other people, and facilitating change in the conduct and understanding of these other people—be they friends, family members, or employers—can be invaluable. The most effective and empowering way in which satisfactory interpersonal reorientation can occur— aside from learning new personal skills—is to assist in changing the social environments of seriously ill people to ones that are more receptive to their needs. In this way, information nights for other people can help to create 'health promoting interpersonal environments' for the person with life-threatening or terminal illness.

7 *Provide relevant referrals.* For some people, the support group alone or regular individual meetings to discuss social issues and problems will not be enough. Serious interpersonal or psychological problems may emerge that might usefully be referred to a consultant psychiatrist, social worker, marriage or family therapist, or perhaps a grief counsellor. Whatever and whoever may be relevant in these cases, it is a practical idea to have access to a local directory of services compiled by the local community health centre, cancer or AIDS council, or government health or welfare department.

8 Finally, the *circulation of information* about common problems that are faced by people who live with chronic or life-threatening illnesses

to media outlets, peak employer and trade union bodies, schools, and churches is a valuable activity. It reminds people that the problems of the seriously ill in our community are everyone's problems and responsibility. It sends the message that a health promoting environment should be sought not just in our hospitals or hospices, but also in our schools and workplaces. Ignorance about death and dying is an enemy of effective and truly compassionate support for those we care about who live with serious illness every day.

To assist reorientation:

1 Provide information.
2 Provide listening and discussion opportunities.
3 Make time regularly.
4 Provide role play opportunities.
5 Provide relevant reference material.
6 Provide information sessions for others.
7 Provide referrals.
8 Circulate information to community.

7

Environmental and Policy Development

Tempora mutantur, et nos mutamur in illis.

The times are changed, and we are changed with them.

Of all the chapters and topics that we have reviewed so far in this book, this chapter is perhaps the most difficult to understand in practical terms. While it is relatively easy to grasp the ideas of health and death education, and to understand their application within support groups, it can be much more difficult to see what one person might do to change the broader environment. The problem of changing professional practices, public policies, or public attitudes towards palliative care can certainly be challenging, but more often it is simply daunting. And yet, it is important that we do not confine ourselves to the easier task of simply providing services to small groups and individuals. To work within a social model of health that is based on the Ottawa Charter is to recognise that working for social change in the broader political and social environment is a normal and proper task to undertake alongside that of direct service provision.

When we speak about wider environmental changes in the context of the goals of a health promoting palliative care, we are really addressing three areas of interest: the enhancement of social supports for those living with serious illness; the encouragement of a reorientation of health services; and the combating of death-denying health policies and practices. But how is one person, or even a small group of busy people, able to identify, initiate, and sustain a modest program aimed at making these kinds of changes? That is the question addressed in this chapter.

The core concerns of environmental and policy development are to:
- enhance broader forms of social support
- encourage a reorientation of health services
- combat death-denying health policies and practices

When I began my research for this chapter, I was struck by the way that the literature seems to divide into two broad categories in the related areas of health promotion, policy development, community development, and palliative care. In other words, there seem to be two kinds of literature written about promoting change in the broader environment. The first kind was characterised by a kind of sociology of policy development that was both grandly abstract and divorced from the everyday world of the practitioner (see, for example, Bunton & Macdonald 1992; Gardner 1992). Here we find analyses of how government develops policies, and theories about the tension, conflict, and sleight of hand demonstrated by competing interest groups in politics, community, and the bureaucratic services. The other type is a kind of push-button literature that is highly practical and highly detailed (see, for example, Wass 1994; Egger et al. 1990). Here we find suggestions about how to write press statements, organise lobby groups, or set up television interviews for one's cause. There is no end to suggestions for attaining public attention—and hence possible policy consideration—for new ideas and practices. In this chapter I will refer to both kinds of literature, but I will dedicate more space to identifying some *basic social and political agendas* that may be adopted—together or individually—in order to encourage changes to the wider policy and practice environment.

There are four separate but linked agendas that need to be discussed: a research agenda, an education and training agenda, a policy-change agenda, and a private-sector support agenda.

Social and political agendas of health promoting palliative care:
- research
- education and training
- policy change
- private-sector support

A RESEARCH AGENDA

There are several good reasons to have a research agenda. We have reviewed the most important elements of these in chapter 2. We will highlight just four of these reasons here in order to revisit and reenforce their relevance to changes in the broader policy and practice environment.

First, and most relevant to direct service provision, is the importance of establishing the credibility and quality of your health promoting service (sometimes referred to as 'quality assurance'). You may need to undertake a needs survey or assessment in relation to the type of service you are thinking of establishing. As well as establishing what the needs of those with serious illness in your area are, such research helps you to determine whether your health promoting service is actually meeting those needs. In other words, to avoid 'flying in the dark', you need to give some thought to evaluation research.

Second, even with the aid of health service surveillance work, there is much we still do not know about the social experience of serious illness from the point of view of those who are actually experiencing it and from the perspective of care-givers. Social research into the experience of living with dying is essential if we are to be able to clearly distinguish the needs of the dying from our own needs. This has not always been clear in the literature written by care-givers. Therefore, research is important in deepening our understanding of what we do, to whom we do it, and why we do it.

Third, research into death and dying remains marginal in relation to mainstream social and health research. There are still only a half-dozen academic journals on death and dying other than the palliative care journals. Worse still is the fact that most writers for palliative care journals refer only to other palliative care journals or to medical or nursing literature, failing to engage or use the social science tradition evident in the older journals of death and dying. This creates an unfortunate impression of the fragmentation and 'ghetto-isation' of a very specialised area. Yet death and dying are not specialised issues. They are part of mainstream and everyday experience. To believe otherwise is to contribute to the widespread social practice of avoiding the importance of death in daily life, and hence to contribute to the marginal position of those with serious illness.

Finally, an important part of influencing public policy concerns lobbying, networking, and creating alliances. However, it is not all politics.
Sometimes evidence for one's views or ideas is required. Research,
when undertaken systematically and with credible designs, is a valuable
tool of leverage in discussions about the need for change. Anyone can
offer groundless opinion—or worse, opinion based on their own
'experience'. Aside from empirical research, there is also the need to
develop the skill of social criticism. The study of public-policy documents and the effective criticism of such documents are important,
perhaps crucial, parts of any health promoting palliative care research
agenda.

Good reasons for having a research agenda:
- quality assurance
- to deepen understanding
- to address 'mainstream' concerns about death and dying
- to create an evidential and critical base for change

Among the many research priorities, I will outline the three most readily identifiable ones in terms of a health promoting palliative care.

The first priority direction for research should be to examine the
experience of living with serious illness from the point of view of
those at the centre of the experience. Most of the research in palliative
care has revolved around care-givers' views of dying and the services
provided to them. Very few articles are based on research with dying
people. Of the articles that deal with the experience of dying, there are
still too few examining differences in conduct and ideas among people
whose identities are influenced by cultures that are not predominantly
English-speaking (Kanitsaki 1998).

There is also still much reluctance and embarrassment surrounding
the study of mystical experiences in the context of dying. Although
there has been a modest tradition of this sort of research among psychologists and a few unusual medical writers, the topic remains highly

contentious. There is no research-oriented reason why this should remain so. A conviction that such experiences do not exist or that they are 'merely' the outcome of a hallucinating, anoxic brain does not itself constitute a good reason for the lack of research in this area. The conviction that schizophrenia is a hallucinatory phenomenon does not impede research into its possible causes or its very real impact on the sufferers and their families. Furthermore, the topic of near-death visions or experiences is one of great interest to most people, including dying people, and for that reason alone, it could arguably be given high priority in any research agenda linked to community concerns.

A study of the relationship between public health and palliative care is also one that can be fruitfully undertaken with minimal professional support. Palliative care is now entering difficult times. Hospice and palliative care services are supported by government financing, and so palliative care faces the same crisis that affects most publicly funded institutions in the Western world, be they schools, universities, hospitals, or welfare providers. If an institution takes the money, it is obliged to take the orders, and the orders that most public institutions are given these days involve cost reduction and rationalisation. What are the options and dangers for palliative care? What are the funding or organisational alternatives?

Although the idea of carrying out empirical research may seem to be beyond the means of those practitioners without additional professional development support, the detailed scrutiny of policy documents is a type of research that is within the reach of any practitioner. The attempt, for example, to offer a thorough critique and outline of alternatives can be research based in that it derives from long and hard thinking, often with others, and from reading broadly on the sociology of health care systems and policy development. Do not dismiss library-based research too quickly.

Whatever your situation, or whatever your specific research interests, you should not believe that social research is beyond your reach or ability. On the subject of methodology, you do not need to conduct surveys or interviews (see Kellehear 1993). Nor do you need to work alone. You do not need to be disempowered by the belief that you have nothing to offer. Everyone is capable of conducting sound research that is both credible and useful to others. The primary requirement is that of being careful and systematic. Prepare for your task by reading widely in the research methodology literature, and work with others. If possible, work with one or two other people who have some research experience. Forming alliances with researchers from other centres, working out who has the skills you need, and searching, identifying, and enlisting the aid of people who have the skills you are lacking are simple, effective networking techniques. Sometimes simply identifying what social research is being conducted into death and dying in your city may lead you to research teams that you may join or assist.

If you live in a small, rural town of, say, 30 000 people or less, there may be no university in your area. In this situation, research that evaluates health services may be more important to you (see, as examples, Wadsworth 1991; Thomas 1992; Sherman & Reid 1994, part 2; Wass 1994, ch. 4; O'Connor & Parker 1995, ch. 4). Unfortunately, the phrase 'evaluation research' produces the same confusion as do terms such as 'data-analysis' or 'semiotics'. Do not be fooled. Evaluation is the code term for a common set of questions: Did the program work (that is, achieve what it set out to do)? Did people in the program find it useful to them? If so, or if not, how do I know this? *That* is evaluation.

There are many ways to find answers to these questions. Ask people what they hope to gain at the beginning of a program (this is sometimes called a 'pre-test') and then ask them at the end whether they felt that they had attained those hopes (sometimes known as a 'post test' or an 'impact evaluation'). You can also keep asking them throughout the program about how they think they are doing (this is often referred to as 'process evaluation'). You can also follow these people up three, six, or nine months later to see if the desired effects have remained with them (sometimes called an 'outcome evaluation'). Methodologically, it might be a good idea to give them a quick questionnaire before and after (a quantitative approach). You might like to sit down and have a long chat with a few of them at regular intervals to find out what they thought about it all (a 'qualitative' approach).

You could even be adventurous and ask those participating in the program how *they* would like the evaluation to be done and what their aims might be in terms of changing the program (rather than simply assuming that you know the criteria for a 'successful' program). The example readings suggested above explore these issues—some more intelligibly than others. Needs surveys, or any recorded information about people's needs when they visit rural services, can contribute valuable demographic and social data to the poor data-bases that most countries have with regard to rural health. Who are the researchers working in rural health? And what do they know about your area, and about death and dying in rural areas? Establishing contact and cooperation with researchers at universities or public-health institutions located elsewhere can be useful and important alliances to make in furthering your research agenda.

EDUCATION AND TRAINING AGENDA

The most important reason for pursuing an education and training agenda as a way of changing the wider social and political environment is the impact it can have on reorienting services. At this stage there are precious few opportunities to learn about health promoting palliative care from institutional sources, and so it is important in terms of individual professional development to learn about the areas most related to these principles.

The idea of 'health promoting settings' is an old one now, and it is useful to learn as much as possible about the principles and cases surrounding this idea for the lessons they may provide for your own practice. If you are a professional working in the health care system, then changing yourself is also a way of changing and reorienting the 'system'. This applies equally, but more obviously, to other people's professional development. We will not reorient health services in public health or palliative care unless we change the way that people in those services see their own services to people who live with serious illness. Education and training, then, is also about networking and hence spreading important ideas within the health system.

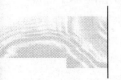

Why have an education and training agenda?
- It is a crucial instrument of change in the professions and therefore the health services.

For the purposes of this section, I will divide the education and training agenda issues into two areas—areas that correspond to the contexts of practitioners working wholly in community settings and those working partly or fully in academic ones.

Community settings

If you are conducting a health promoting palliative care program in a setting that has no formal contact with a university or technical college, there are still ways that you might influence the education and training of other professionals. Remember that if you are running or thinking of conducting a health promoting palliative care service, you have, *ipso facto*, reoriented health services by your very existence. Change is not just 'out there' but 'inside here'; it is part of you and what you do. Let me begin, then, with *your own education and training possibilities.*

You may begin by identifying and seeking out the academic or university public-health departments in your city. Sometimes these will be part of schools of medicine or nursing. At other times they will be 'free-standing' departments that belong to generic health science faculties. Most of these departments will have a staff seminar program that runs over the length of the year. Most of them are delighted (even desperate) to have visitors attending their meetings. Phone the relevant department and ask to be placed on its mailing list so that you can decide which seminars will be of use to you in deepening and broadening your understanding of health promotion.

Another alternative is to consider asking some of the staff in those university departments to come to your workplace to offer a seminar or presentation on public-health or health promotion matters. Sometimes your workplace may have staff-development money to pay for these visits. If not, think about an 'honorarium'—a token gift of $100 or so, which shows the recipients that you value their effort and help. At other times, you may ask them if they will come to talk to your group without a fee but promise them good coffee and an attentive audience—both increasingly rare commodities on university campuses these days.

Aside from seminars to attend, one may think about short courses. These can often be found advertised in public-health journals or the professional journals of health carers. The *Higher Education Supplement* of the *Australian* newspaper and the *Campus Review* newspaper often advertise these short courses too. And do not just think in terms of health promotion or public health. Many good short courses are run for new researchers on research design and data-analysis. But do not enrol in short courses on research unless you are actually about to embark on your own research. The information and learning gained in short courses is not often retained unless you use it quickly. Few lessons remain intact without practice.

If you are sceptical of the benefits of short courses (ones that run for one or two weeks or over a weekend), think about enrolling in one whole semester-length subject at university or technical college. These are 'non-degree' subjects which you can attend alongside degree students. There will be class-attendance requirements (lectures and tutorials), regular assignments, and maybe exams. Most universities are happy to enrol 'non-degree' students, also sometimes known as 'miscellaneous enrolments'. A fee is usually charged.

Staff exchanges, as mentioned in chapter 2, are also useful ways to learn. Palliative care staff might arrange for temporary exchanges with staff in public- or community-health workplaces as a way of familiarising themselves with the language, concepts, and practices of those in health promotion and public health.

Finally, if none of these options are realistic for you or your colleagues, a reading group is also a useful way to maintain staff development and enhance education and training with respect to health promoting palliative care. Many workplaces have a 'journal club', where staff members are asked to read one recently published article and another staff member is asked to lead the discussion about that piece. This method of staff development can be used to get the most out of books and articles on health promotion and social studies of death and dying.

As for encouraging the ideas of health promoting palliative care in the *education and training of other people*, many of the suggestions just reviewed work equally well. Instead of attending seminars in university departments of public health (where they are unlikely to run courses on topics such as palliative care), you might conduct and advertise seminars for others on health promoting palliative care. The public-health professionals in your local area may be intrigued with the combination of these terms ('health promotion' and 'palliative care') alone.

Aside from conducting your own seminars, you might consider volunteering to offer a presentation on your work ideas and practices to the local university public-health or palliative care seminar series. Such a presentation does not have to be highly theoretical. Practical knowledge is important knowledge too. Its presentation usefully challenges the masculinist and unhelpful idea that the only worthwhile knowledge derives from abstract (theoretical) and distant (objective) reflections on experience. Other staff from local palliative care services may be interested in the idea of health promoting palliative care, or perhaps your version of it. These are ideal forums for the exchange of ideas, and can create networking possibilities for research and writing collaborations with colleagues.

Rather than enrolling in single subjects at university or technical college, you could offer single subjects yourself, targeted at health professions, at the local college of adult education. If no such institution exists in your area, you could still run fee-paying short courses for interested professionals as part of your own drive to promote staff development in this area.

Rather than simply asking other agencies to allow you or your colleagues to spend time at their community health agency, you might invite other public-health professionals to come and work at your agency in order to learn how health promotion principles can work in a palliative care setting and practice. Even if there is little time or resources for such exchanges, it may still be possible to encourage 'site visits' and joint agency 'lunches' to exchange ideas, resources, and—perhaps in the future—staff.

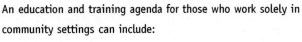

An education and training agenda for those who work solely in community settings can include:
- reading groups
- site visits
- staff exchanges
- seminar attendance or presentations
- short course offerings
- single-subject tertiary-level enrolments

Academic settings

I will briefly devote some space here to strategies that colleagues in the academy can use to promote an education and training agenda for health promotion in palliative care. Most of the following possibilities apply to curriculum change and should be familiar to most academic readers, but in case some readers are not aware of one or two options, I will summarise all of these possibilities.

The most obvious way to introduce a subject in health promoting palliative care in any undergraduate or graduate program is to offer that subject as an elective. Because professional degree programs in nursing, medicine, or social work are highly structured programs, the elective offerings are good ways to attract interested students. This is, of course, the main limitation to elective offerings—they are not part of the mainstream, compulsory offerings that are presented to students.

Existing 'core' subjects in palliative care or public health may also be redesigned to incorporate sections dedicated to a study of health promoting palliative care. Some class assignments in health promoting palliative care may also be submitted as part of students' compulsory written or oral work. At the very least, some lectures on the relevance of health promoting palliative care to public-health or health care professional services will be useful.

Finally, a specialised graduate program, such as a diploma or certificate course, may be offered in health promoting palliative care. This might involve a curriculum made up of subjects dedicated to reviewing and examining the various health promotion and research strategies in the context of the broad aims of hospice and palliative care. A subject examining the historical links between public health and palliative care would make a sound first orientation subject.

These suggestions largely assume that academic departments have the resources to offer new elective subjects, or even that they are able to be so ambitious as to offer new graduate programs. These are not wise assumptions to make these days. If you have neither the staff nor the funding to provide such offerings, what are the other options?

First, interdepartmental links can be forged so that existing subjects in health promotion offered in the health sciences area might be made available to students outside that area. Students in nursing or pastoral care, for example, may be encouraged to take an elective subject in health promotion. The direct relevance of a generalist health promotion curriculum to palliative care may not be specific enough without some modification to the assignment tasks. Staff from different professional areas participating in this educational and training collaboration may require their own students in those subjects to receive different, more palliative care oriented, examination. This option can equally apply to academics in public health who, in their turn, may permit their students to enrol in palliative care courses that are strong in 'psycho-social' content and to sit examinations that require health promotion input. In cases where the one university does not have significant and relevant departments of nursing, medicine, and health promotion, and where such cross-area collaborations are not possible (or politically and administratively achievable), the facility of 'complementary enrolment' may overcome the problem. In this case, students may enrol in subjects offered by another university, on a one-off basis, which will be counted towards their degrees at their 'home' university. This is particularly convenient if there are more than one or two universities in your home town or city. In rural areas, where often there is only one university operating, complementary enrolment may still be possible through a major distance-education provider. These are options that are worth exploring in an academic world of shrinking resources, in which successful course offerings result only from being smarter and more strategic in one's thinking.

Finally, it must be noted that all of the education and training strategies described in relation to community settings also apply to those of us in the academy. Reading groups, site visits, seminar attendance and presentations, and short-course offerings and attendance can be equally useful parts of an educational agenda for those in the academy. Furthermore, staff exchanges can be facilitated by colleagues in public health or palliative care who wish to devote part or all of their study leave to spending time in each other's areas. Instead of palliative care academics spending all of their study leave in palliative care departments at other universities, they may spend some time in a public health or a specifically health promotion oriented department—for example, a department of health education.

POLICY CHANGE AGENDA

Until now, we have devoted all the discussion in this chapter to a research agenda and to an education and training agenda dedicated to *change*—change to enable public health and palliative care workers to exchange ideas and to see the value of knowing each other better. And if such exchanges were more common, their impact might also directly affect how well we are able to create supportive environments for those with serious illness through our professional services and offerings to them.

A policy change and private-sector agenda, though, has an additional objective: *resistance*. Both palliative care and public health have one further characteristic in common with each other: they both have a distinguished history of reforming a stubborn and entrenched status quo (Daly et al. 1997). Today, the need for resistance and change in palliative care has not been as great since the early years of hospice care. Judy Parker and Sanchia Aranda (1998)—and with one or two exceptions, most of the contributors in their collection of essays—lament the changes that are sweeping the health care system and that now threaten the original ideals of hospice care (see especially Rumbold 1998). The threat of 'mainstreaming', particularly into acute care services (often referred to as 'integrating services'), means the re-emergence of territorial disputes between different professions over control of resources, team leadership, and preferred research paradigms.

The rise of 'managed care' in countries such as Australia and the USA, for example, means that 'content-free' management principles threaten to undermine and overtake the traditional territorial disputes between the professions. The idea that most professionals are partisan in their understanding of patient or client needs, and that a 'manager' can oversee the larger requirements and, at times, even administer a health care budget to provide overall care, has had two detrimental effects on service provision. First, interest in managed care has increased tension and competition between professions, as each vies against the other in a public-relations exercise to convince governments that it, rather than the other professions, is better equipped to undertake 'case management'. Professional rivalry, rather than cooperation, has been the net result here. Second, the lack of adequate resistance to this latest wave of economic rationalism and new managerialism has disempowered professionals, leading them to inadvertently accept a bureaucratic, managerialist response to health care. Managed care can undermine the philosophy and ideals of interdisciplinary team care and management. This is particularly dangerous to, and undermining of, the original holistic ideals of hospice and palliative care. A policy agenda of any health promoting palliative care, therefore, might usefully include resistance to these specific developments.

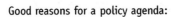

Good reasons for a policy agenda:
- It promotes health promotion in palliative care policy.
- It promotes interdisciplinary cooperation and resource sharing.
- It resists current changes that undermine hospice and palliative care ideals.
- It resists changes that reduce professional cooperation and cooperative team management.

What strategies might be undertaken? First, a long-term campaign of publications is important. Contributing articles to journals—both peer-review and opinion-based journals—is important and has value in creating discussion, generating criticism, and forcing yourself and others to explain and be accountable. For example, for a long time now, governments have stressed the importance of evaluation in any kind of service provision. In that context, it will be important to encourage ongoing evaluation of managed care beyond the initial 'trials' that are used to herald the arrival of such systems of care. The question of the validity, reliability, and relevance to clients of any evaluation design for such managed care programs needs ongoing monitoring and scrutiny. But this surveillance notwithstanding, we must not be falsely led into assuming that good evaluation results mean that the philosophy or service approach is superior to previous or alternative health care approaches. Managed care comes at a time when public spending on education, health, and welfare is in crisis, and we must not forget that many new models of care result from a desire to contain costs rather than to improve services. At the very least, the major intellectual and policy problem for even the most compassionate policy-maker these days seems to be about merely maintaining current services (and current service gaps) with less expenditure.

Second, forming alliances is also an important strategy for influencing policy. Once again, it can be useful for palliative care workers to form alliances with community-development and public health groups, not simply to draw on their more participatory ideas about service provision, but also to benefit from their experience in social action. Professional associations can also be useful places to form alliances. Some professionals argue that their associations are the breeding grounds for the most conservative members of their profession. Whether or not that observation is true, it is certainly an ahistorical and non-sociological view of associations. Most professional associations have, at some time in their history, or over some issue or another, become active agents of change. Furthermore, an unsympathetic professional association executive can only be changed by filling the positions on that executive with like-minded colleagues. Staying away from that professional association will ensure that you do not take the first step towards achieving that goal. Forging alliances with other disaffected groups will also be important in combating the impression that resistance to undesirable changes is confined to marginal groups. Since palliative care is an interdisciplinary field and the current changes sweeping the health care system affect many people outside palliative care, all the professions involved and their associations are potential allies.

Third, conference presentations in professional and academic forums, although of limited use in policy development, should be undertaken where possible. However, presentations to consumer groups and to business organisations will be more important. Service organisations are always interested to hear from professionals, and these settings are well attended by the business community.

Fourth, political lobbying is an important activity, and one that should be undertaken regularly. This 'lobbying'—the petitioning or 'begging' for help—can be performed in a dignified manner at any professional association, state or federal department of health services, and also your local politician. Do not underestimate the power of a personal visit. All unpopular political and administrative decisions are made much easier by having less personal contact with those whom they affect.

There is a prevalent view about today that argues that we must make do with what we receive (note the alarming similarity with the language of a well-known 'grace before meals' prayer). In this way, the times are changed, and we are steadily, gradually, imperceptibly, and incrementally made to change with them. A certain acceptance, if not complacency, develops around changes that we feel we do not control, and rationalisations such as the one above take hold.

But simply accepting and 'making do' conveys an unhelpful and false message that the only meaningful and effective action to be taken is action among ourselves—'real' power lies with others. However, political power, and hence the impetus for change, does not only lie with others—it lies with ourselves and with our allies. This is what John Catford (1992, p. xi) means when he argues that 'health promoters need to show that they are actively working "upstream"'. To reorient health services, and to provide a more supportive environment for users of palliative care services, we must reorient key decision-makers.

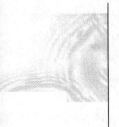

A policy change agenda includes:

- publishing activity
- activity with professional associations
- public presentations—to colleagues, but also consumers and business audiences
- political lobbying
- the encouragement of participatory and equitable forms of cooperation and management

Finally, the rise of professional rivalry and tensions over leadership, expert knowledge, preferred research designs, or resources must be actively resisted if we are to avoid a return to the unhelpful interprofessional slanging matches of the 1970s. Charges of 'medical dominance', or the equally inflammatory idea that nurses are somehow 'less expert', will only encourage professional 'tribalism' at a time when everyone's 'village' is being sacked and plundered. Remember that in a time of diminishing resources, those with less sociological imagination about the sources of their troubles turn on each other.

The way forward is actively to encourage *closer* research and educational links; genuine sharing of resources in collaborative research and service initiatives; more participatory forms of management; and the active promotion of analyses that identify the common problems and the barriers to their solution. In this context, we cannot fully separate the policy-change agenda from a private-sector support agenda because the government drives most of the retrograde policy changes. It is able to sanction these changes and to exercise its powers through the funding ties it has to the different services. This is the difficult and complex problem to which we now turn.

PRIVATE-SECTOR SUPPORT AGENDA

There are several important reasons why a private-sector support strategy is important, both generally and specifically, as an aid to a policy-change agenda. First, the private sector is an alternative source of funding, and it also has the support of the public's interest. There are few people who have not somehow been touched by cancer or HIV in their own lives, and they are usually more than willing to help out in whatever small way they can. Few people have been untouched by serious illness or death. They will listen to appeals to help a palliative care service. As an alternative source of financial resources, the private sector can facilitate an alternative political (and hence 'power') base by allowing you greater control of your own research, policy, and service design. Private-sector financial support can enhance or create an ability to resist retrograde service and policy directions within your service that might be tied to government funding. Independent funding can assist in providing quasi or total independence from those requirements. In this way, an alternative resource allocation can be a powerful form of resistance.

Second, businesses, particularly large businesses, have stronger political links to local, state, and federal governments than do small palliative care services, and so links to those businesses can supply not only financial support, but also de facto political support. Sponsors can act as other 'courts of appeal'. In other words, if State bureaucracies require changes to your service that you consider to be highly compromising, sympathetic sponsors can make their own displeasure over those changes known in other political arenas. Relationships with private-sector sponsors can be useful and valuable political alliances, if not in changing government policy, then at least in helping to resist some of it.

Third, although service providers are often required to boast about or publicise the names of their sponsors, it is also true that sponsors boast about or publicise those services that they have chosen to support. In this way, private-sector support can provide different but important alternative avenues of advertising and support in creating public awareness of palliative care services. Creating private-sector links maximises effective public awareness.

Finally, although public-sector workers have traditionally been shy of relationships with big business, remember that health promotion is everyone's responsibility and not just the individual's (see chapter 1). The private sector, including business interests, is an important part of any sociological or political definition of 'everyone'.

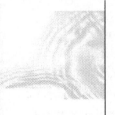

> Good reasons for a private-sector support agenda:
> - It provides greater independence in controlling the philosophy and practice of service provision, research, and policy.
> - It provides an alternative and greater source of political support.
> - It maximises effective public awareness.
> - Health promotion is everyone's responsibility—not just the public sector's.

Although it is easy to see how important it is to develop a private-sector support strategy, some may ask whether this strategy might actually help government to avoid its own responsibilities towards palliative care. I think the answer to that criticism is that such a strategy *can* encourage governments to avoid their responsibilities, but on the other hand, it might not do this and ought not to do this. When approached for support, many potential donors and sponsors will ask why the government is not supporting the service. Obviously, for many palliative care or health promotion services, government support will be in place, but you will be seeking additional support—maybe for the health promoting palliative care functions. Other groups or individuals may be starting with no support at all. This is a perfect time to educate potential sponsors. In these moments, you can discuss the original hospice ideals or those of health promotion through the philosophical prism of the Ottawa Charter, and describe what you see as the threats to these ideals. Depending on the sophistication of your own analyses, these ideals may be discussed in the context of the gradual collapse of the public sector in the last thirty years or so. Whatever the topic, the policy implications of shrinking resources might be explained so that political pressures might be brought to bear on governments whether you are successful in gaining financial support or not. Already many companies are complaining about the increasing number of sponsorship requests that they are receiving each year and are wondering where this might end. These are healthy and promising questions for governments and business to ask each other as we enter a new century.

So what strategies might be employed to encourage private-sector support? There are three principal strategies for developing a private-sector support agenda. They are the enlistment of media support, the enlistment of private health and social-services support, and the attraction of corporate sponsorship and donations.

The enlistment of media support can perform three functions. First, the use of the media can help disseminate criticism and research findings. Governments are not concerned about adverse research or policy findings in peer-reviewed journals. Such criticism can be viewed, as former Australian prime minister Paul Keating once observed, as similar to 'being flogged by a warm lettuce' (Bookman Press 1992). Controversial or highly critical findings must make their way into the popular media—newspapers, radio, or television—if they are to have any potential to change policy.

The media can also be valuable in publicising your program's activities. In this way, the media are important in creating public awareness of health promoting palliative care. Often radio stations and local newspapers, even large city dailies, will have community notices that will help to publicise the work of your program. Community radio should also be considered as a potential avenue of support in these areas.

Finally, self-referrals may readily come from ordinary people if they know of the service you are providing. Bequests, and other donations from individuals, will only flow from actual experience of your service or from knowing about the good work provided by your service. The cooperation of the local radio or newspaper networks in your area will be crucial in cultivating this source of clientele and increasing public awareness.

It will be important to enlist the help of private health and social services, not only because it is important that both private and public providers support the ideal of health promoting palliative care, but also because such help will sometimes be important in the actual provision of services. It will often be important to provide legal, funeral, or financial-counselling support and information, and these can rarely be provided without the cooperation of the relevant business sectors. Furthermore, private hospitals and health insurance companies may also be eager to learn of innovations directly from innovative providers and can assist in the provision of physical spaces, equipment, or advertising in exchange for some staff training or support in the health promoting palliative care area. Health insurance companies have an obvious interest in both public health and palliative care, and will be important potential sponsors as well.

The attraction of sponsorships and donations should not be seen in purely financial terms, although this will be very important. It is important to solicit financial support for administration or direct service costs. However, sponsors can also assist with the donation of equipment or the advertising and publicity needs of your program. They may also provide small sponsorships of lunches for professional meetings, of research, or of conferences. You need to think in terms of how your activities will help the publicity agenda of your sponsor, because it is a fact of life that sponsorship is a commercial activity as well as a philanthropic one.

Finally, some companies may not be able to assist financially at all, but may be quite sympathetic to the ideals of a health promoting palliative care. These corporations may be interested in lending their name and considerable corporate reputation to submissions to hearings organised by government to consider policy issues. Imagine if a critical submission about current palliative care services came not only from Tobruk Community Health Centre, but also IBM, Coca-Cola, and BHP. Any reply or response to the ideas in that submission would need to take account of counter responses by those companies. It is an interesting thought, is it not?

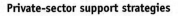

Private-sector support strategies

Enlist the media to:

- disseminate criticism and research findings
- create public awareness
- generate self referrals

Enlist private health and social services to:

- support health promoting palliative care services
- help with sponsorships

Attract sponsorship and donations to:

- help offset administration and direct service costs
- sponsor research and conferences
- support policy submissions and comment

These private-sector support strategies perform two crucial functions of any health promoting palliative care service. First, such strategies, as methods of community development, help to create an environment where subsequent policy development may favour the work and ideals of health promoting palliative care. They may do so by enlisting the support of two of the most powerful influences in any community: the media and the corporate sector. Whether one favours a pluralist, an élites, or a structural, Marxist, or corporatist view of the policy process (Gardner & Barraclough 1992), such alliances will be crucial to the politics of change and resistance that are so central now to the concerns of palliative care—health promoting or any other kind.

Second, all the above social and political agendas help to create a broader social and political environment of support. People who confront the problems of living with serious illnesses will do so with a greater likelihood that the responsibility for the support and alleviation of those problems will be shared by all of us. In this sociological way, these agendas create supportive environments that go beyond the limited world of support groups. The likelihood of meeting the Ottawa Charter's goals of reorienting health services, of creating truly supportive environments, and of strengthening community action for those living with dying only becomes a genuine possibility within the contexts of these wider agendas. This is the personal and public face, and the responsibility, of all health promoting palliative care.

Concluding Thoughts

Nowadays, as we move into the new millennium, we are frequently prompted to reflect on the old one. Philippe Aries (1974) writes of a time in the Middle Ages when a dying person was someone who was at the very centre of his or her social activity. In other words, Aries describes a time when dying people controlled and regulated the social activity around them, and the primary activity around them was often religious. This depiction stands in stark contrast to the picture of the dying person throughout most of the twentieth century. Here Aries, with countless other social observers of our time, describes the disempowered dying person of modernity. Removed from the surroundings of his or her home and the familiar faces of friends, the dying person of the twentieth century has often been an institutionalised victim of stigma and embarrassment. The primary activity around the dying person has been medical. Simple knowledge about impending death has been communicated by a nod of the head or a press of the hands. Sometimes it has not been communicated at all. In this way, dying people in the twentieth century have represented a dark opposite of their counterparts in earlier centuries. The hospice and palliative care movement, together with a new groundswell of academic, professional, and popular literature in the 1970s, began to rebuild and restore the fallen, disempowered, and lonely figure of the dying person.

We will not return to the 'romantic' times described by Aries because, to some extent, the picture of the autonomous and controlling dying person was somewhat elusive even then. The severity of the symptomatology of infectious disease, or the sheer suddenness of death in medieval times, makes Aries's descriptions more ideal than realistic in most cases. It is true that there is ample evidence of segregation and rejection of dying people in the course that clinical work has taken over the twentieth century. However, there is equal evidence of a desire to forge new and compassionate ways to conceptualise and treat the dying person, aside from seeing the person merely as an 'incurable case'. There have been many practitioners who have resisted the idea of dying as failure and who have sought instead to understand dying as living. This has been the main message and the central assumption of modern hospice and palliative care.

Despite that consistently held ideal, however, much of the thrust of our attention has remained devoted to concerns about physical, end-stage care. One can still see this in the preponderance of articles on symptom control, particularly pain control. The work in this area grows stronger and more systematic each year. But, sadly, the literature on what has come to be known, somewhat confusingly, as 'psycho-social' care seems not to have grown in a commensurate and equally credible way. Each year, we witness new programs that are unable or unwilling to acknowledge the different and important differences in the psychological and social care of people with life-threatening or terminal illnesses. Such conceptual poverty does not augur well for the parallel ability to observe and understand these distinctions in real people. A stronger theoretical basis for the care of people's social and psychological needs has been required for some time now.

Health promoting palliative care offers a model of social care based on critical and participatory principles drawn from both palliative care and health promotion as endorsed by the World Health Organization. Together these fields provide us with a promising way forward, rooted in a commitment to people's social needs, and with a view to helping facilitate a new way of living and dying in the new millennium. 'Dying well' is no longer simply a question of the patient being in control or the doctor being in control; nor is it simply an issue of dying at home or in an institution. Living and dying can move towards a participatory model of health care that might involve multiple sites and different decision-makers, at different times. But most of the time, we can make decisions together, as clinicians and as people who will die. We can share the doubts and explore the issues, consulting with each other. All journeys of illness involve changing stories, in which the key players or the powerful players change places, and maybe more than once. And this is how it should be.

It is true that a health promoting palliative care is a style of palliative care that returns our interest to the early period of dying. But it is much more than this. It also focuses our attention on the worthy practice principles of participation, support, and consultation right up to the end of life. Although these are the core values of health promotion, and of palliative care, they are not the number-one priority of policies motivated by economic rationalism and the new managerialism associated with it. In this way, health promoting palliative care pits the two most powerful and reformist traditions of health care against the current movement towards undermining quality care for the chronically ill.

Finally, a health promoting palliative care philosophy renews our practical commitment to the social side of life—in the very person before us, and in the wider society to which he or she belongs. Health promoting palliative care offers an opportunity to deepen our understanding of the finer distinctions of human need that go beyond the body—the needs of the spirit and mind, and of the social world that cradles and nurtures them both. Only in this renewed commitment to the social will palliative care be able to deliver to successive generations in the new millennium the twin offerings of both bread and hyacinths.

Bibliography

Anderson, P. 1991, *Affairs in Order: A Complete Resource Guide to Death and Dying*, Macmillan, New York.

Aries, P. 1974, *Western Attitudes toward Death*, Johns Hopkins University Press, London.

Bander, P. 1973, *Voices from the Tapes: Recordings from the Other World*, Drake, New York.

Barouh, G. 1992, *Support Groups: The Human Face of the HIV/AIDS Epidemic*, Long Island Association for AIDS Care Inc., New York.

Basil, R. (ed.) 1989, *Not Necessarily the New Age: Critical Essays*, Prometheus, New York.

Becker, E. 1973, *The Denial of Death*, Collier–Macmillan, New York.

Birrell, F. & Lucas, F. L. (eds) 1930, *The Art of Dying: An Anthology*, Hogarth Press, London.

Blackmore, S. 1993, *Dying to Live: Science and the Near-Death Experience*, Grafton, London.

Bookman Press (ed.) 1992, *Paul Keating's Book of Insults*, Bookman Press, Melbourne.

Brown, N. O. 1968, *Life against Death: The Psychoanalytic Meaning of History*, Sphere, London.

Buckman, R. 1996, *What You Really Need to Know about Cancer: A Comprehensive Guide for Patients and their Families*, Hodder & Stoughton, Sydney.

Bunston, T., Mings, D., Mackie, A., & Jones, D. 1995, 'Facilitating Hopefulness: The Determinants of Hope', *Journal of Psychosocial Oncology*, vol. 13, no. 4, pp. 79–103.

Bunton, R. & Macdonald, G. (eds) 1992, *Health Promotion: Disciplines and Diversity*, Routledge, London.

Bunton, R., Nettleton, S., & Burrows, R. 1995, *The Sociology of Health Promotion: Critical Analyses of Consumption, Lifestyle and Risk*, Routledge, London.

Camus, A. 1961, *The Outsider*, Penguin Books, Harmondsworth.

Carpenter, J. P. 1977, *The Screwdriver (Does It or Doesn't It?)*, Arizona State Museum Library, University of Arizona, Tucson.

Catford, J. 1992, 'Vital Signs of Health Promotion', in R. Bunton & G. Macdonald (eds), *Health Promotion: Disciplines and Diversity*, Routledge, London, pp. x–xii.

Charles, K., Sellick, S. M., Montesanto, B., & Mohide, E. A. 1996, 'Priorities of Cancer Survivors Regarding Psychosocial Needs', *Journal of Psychosocial Oncology*, vol. 14, no. 2, pp. 57–72.

Charmaz, K., Howarth, G., & Kellehear, A. (eds) 1997, *The Unknown Country: Death in Australia, Britain, and the USA*, Macmillan, Basingstoke.

Chiverton, E. 1997, 'Social Support within the Context of Life Threatening Illness', *International Journal of Palliative Care*, vol. 3, pp. 107–10.

Clark, D. 1994, 'At the Crossroads: Which Direction for the Hospices?', *Palliative Medicine*, vol. 8, pp. 1–3.

Cohn-Sherbock, D. & Lewis, C. (eds) 1995, *Beyond Death: Theological and Philosophical Reflections on Life after Death*, Macmillan, Basingstoke.

Colquhoun, D. 1991, 'Health Education in Australia', *Annual Review of Health Social Sciences*, vol. 1, pp. 7–29.

Daly, J., Kellehear, A., & Gliksman, M. 1997, *The Public Health Researcher: A Methodological Guide*, Oxford University Press, Melbourne.

Dessaix, R. 1996, *Night Letters: A Journey through Switzerland and Italy*, Macmillan, Sydney.

Dignan, M. & Carr, P. 1987, *Program Planning for Health Education and Health Promotion*, Lea & Febiger, Philadelphia.

Dinnage, R. 1992, *The Ruffian on the Stair: Reflections on Death*, Penguin Books, Harmondsworth.

Doyle, D., Hanks, G. W. C., & MacDonald, N. (eds) 1993, *Oxford Textbook of Palliative Medicine*, Oxford University Press, Oxford.

Dudgeon, D. J., Raubertas, R. F., Doerner, K., O'Connor, T., Tobin, M., & Rosenthal, S. N. 1995, 'When Does Palliative Care Begin? A Needs Assessment of Cancer Patients with Recurrent Disease', *Journal of Palliative Care*, vol. 11, pp. 5–9.

Eddy, J. M. & Alles, W. F. 1983, *Death Education*, C.V. Mosby & Co., London.

Eddy, J. M. & Duff, P. E. 1986, 'Should Values Clarification be a Goal of Death Education?', *Death Studies*, vol. 10, pp. 155–63.

Edgar, L., Remmer, J., Rosberger, Z., & Rapkin, B. 1996, 'An Oncology Volunteer Support Organisation: The Benefits and Fit within the Health Care System', *Psycho-oncology*, vol. 5, pp. 331–41.

Egger, G., Spark, R., & Lawson, J. 1990, *Health Promotion Strategies and Methods*, McGraw-Hill, Sydney.

Elliot, G. 1972, *Twentieth Century Book of the Dead*, Allen Lane, London.

Ellis, D. J. 1978, *The Mediumship of the Tape Recorder*, Society for Psychical Research, London.

Enright, D. J. (ed.) 1987, *The Oxford Book of Death*, Oxford University Press, Oxford.

Fawzy, F. I., Fawzy, N. W., Arndt, L. A., & Pasnau, R. O. 1995, 'Critical Review of Psychosocial Interventions in Cancer Care', *Archives of General Psychiatry*, vol. 52, pp. 100–13.

Finucane, R. C. 1996, *Ghosts: Appearances of the Dead and Cultural Transformation*, Prometheus, New York.

Fobair, P. 1997, 'Cancer Support Groups and Group Therapies: Part 1. Historical and Theoretical Background and Research on Effectiveness', *Journal of Psychosocial Oncology*, vol. 15, no. 1, pp. 63–81.

Foley, F. J., Flannery, J., Graydon, D., Flintoft, G., & Cook, D. 1995, 'AIDS Palliative Care—Challenging the Palliative Paradigm', *Journal of Palliative Care*, vol. 11, pp. 19–22.

Frankel, V. 1973, *The Doctor and the Soul*, Penguin Books, Harmondsworth.

French, J. & Adams, L. 1986, 'From Analysis to Synthesis: Theories of Health Education', *Health Education Journal*, vol. 45, no. 2, pp. 71–4.

Freud, S. 1915, 'Thoughts for the Times on War and Death', in J. Strachey (ed.), *Standard Edition of the Complete Psychological Works of Sigmund Freud*, vol. 14, Hogarth Press, London, pp. 275–300.

—— 1971 (1920), *Beyond the Pleasure Principle*, Hogarth Press, London.

Gallop, G. (with W. Proctor) 1982, *Adventures in Immortality*, Souvenir Press, London.

Gardner, H. (ed.) 1992, *Health Policy: Development, Implementation and Evaluation in Australia*, Longman Cheshire, Melbourne.

Gardner, H. & Barraclough, S. 1992, 'The Policy Process', in H. Gardner (ed.), *Health Policy: Development, Implementation and Evaluation in Australia*, Longman Cheshire, Melbourne, pp. 3–28.

Glasser, B. G. & Strauss, A. L. 1968, *Time for Dying*, Aldine, Chicago.

Goffman, E. 1974, *Stigma*, Penguin Books, Harmondsworth.

Goode, A. (ed.) 1992, *More Great Working Dog Stories*, ABC Books, Sydney.

Gotay, C. C. 1991, 'Accrual to Cancer Clinical Trials: Directions from the Research Literature', *Social Science and Medicine*, vol. 36, no. 12, pp. 569–77.

Grande, G. E., Todd, C. J., & Barclay, S. I. G. 1997, 'Support Needs in the Last Year of Life: Patient and Carer Dilemmas', *Palliative Medicine*, vol. 11, pp. 202–8.

Grande, G. E., Todd, C. J., Barclay, S. I. G., & Doyle, J. H. 1996, 'What Terminally Ill Patients Value in the Support Provided by GPs, District and Macmillan Nurses', *International Journal of Palliative Nursing*, vol. 2, pp. 138–43.

Greenberg, J. S. 1988, *Health Education: Learner Centred Instructional Strategies*, Wm C. Brown Publishers, Dubuque, Ia.

Guggenheim, B. & Guggenheim, J. 1996, *Hello from Heaven*, Thorsons, London.

Hann, D. E., Oxman, T. E., Ahles, T. A., Furstenberg, C. T., & Stuke, T.A. 1995, 'Social Support Adequacy and Depression in Older Patients with Metastatic Cancer', *Psycho-oncology*, vol. 4, pp. 213–21.

Haug, F. 1992, *Beyond Female Masochism: Memory Work and Politics*, Verso, London.

Herman, J. 1995, 'The Demise of the Randomised Control Trial', *Journal of Clinical Epidemiology*, vol. 48, pp. 985–8.

Hick, J. 1976, *Death and Eternal Life*, Collins, London.

Hodder, P. & Turley, A. 1989, *The Creative Option of Palliative Care: A Manual for Health Professionals*, Melbourne City Mission, Melbourne.

Iacovino, V. & Reesor, K. 1997, 'Literature on Interventions to Address Cancer Patients' Psychosocial Needs: What Does It Tell Us?', *Journal of Psychosocial Oncology*, vol. 15, no. 2, pp. 47–71.

Johnston, G. & Abraham, C. 1995, 'The WHO Objectives for Palliative Care: To What Extent Are We Achieving them?', *Palliative Medicine*, vol. 9, pp. 123–37.

Jones, C. 1989, *The Search for Meaning*, ABC Books, Sydney.

Judd, F. K., Cockram, A., Mijch, A., & McKenzie, D. 1997, 'Liaison Psychiatry in an HIV/AIDS Unit', *Australian and New Zealand Journal of Psychiatry*, vol. 31, no. 3, pp. 391–7.

Kane, J. 1991, *Be Sick Well: A Healthy Approach to Chronic Illness*, New Harbinger Publications, Oakland, Calif.

Kanitsaki, O. 1998, 'Palliative Care and Cultural Diversity', in J. Parker & S. Aranda (eds), *Palliative Care: Explorations and Challenges*, MacLennan & Petty, Sydney, pp. 32–45.

Katcher, A. & Beck, A. (eds) 1983, *New Perspectives on our Lives with Companion Animals*, University of Philadelphia Press, Philadelphia.

Kearl, M. 1989, *Endings: A Sociology of Death and Dying*, Oxford University Press, New York.

Kearney, M. 1992, 'Palliative Medicine: Just Another Speciality?', *Palliative Medicine*, vol. 6, pp. 39–46.

Keizer, B. 1996, *Dancing with Mr D: Notes on Life and Death*, Doubleday, London.

Kellehear, A. 1990, *Dying of Cancer: The Final Year of Life*, Harwood Academic Publishers, London.

—— 1993, *The Unobtrusive Researcher: A Guide to Methods*, Allen & Unwin, Sydney.

—— 1994, 'The Social Inequality of Dying', in C. Waddell & A. Peterson (eds), *Just Health: Inequality in Illness, Care and Prevention*, Churchill Livingstone, Melbourne, pp. 181–9.

—— 1996, *Experiences Near Death: Beyond Medicine and Religion*, Oxford University Press, New York.

Kellehear, A. & Fook, J. 1989, 'Sociological Factors in Death Denial by the Terminally Ill', in J. L. Sheppard (ed.), *Advances in Behavioural Medicine*, vol. 6, Cumberland College of Health Sciences, Sydney, pp. 527–37.

—— 1997, 'Lassie Come Home: A Study of "Lost Pet" Notices', *Omega*, vol. 34, no. 3, pp. 191–202.

Kelly, B., Dunne, M., Raphael, B., Buckham, C., Zournazi, A., Smith, S., et al. 1991, 'Relationships between Mental Adjustment to HIV Diagnosis, Psychological Morbidity and Sexual Behaviour', *British Journal of Clinical Psychology*, vol. 30, pp. 370–2.

Kickbush, I. 1989, 'Self-Care in Health Promotion', *Social Science and Medicine*, vol. 29, pp. 125–30.

Koutroulis, G. 1996, 'Memory-Work: Process, Practice and Pitfalls', in D. Colquhoun & A. Kellehear (eds), *Health Research in Practice*, vol. 2, *Personal Experiences, Public Issues*, Chapman & Hall, London, pp. 95–113.

Kubler-Ross, E. 1978, *To Live until We Say Good-bye*, Prentice-Hall, Englewood Cliffs, NJ.

Kung, H. 1984, *Eternal Life?*, Collins, London.

LaGrand, L. E. 1997, *After Death Communication*, Llewellyn Publications, St Paul, Minn.

Lee, L. & Lee, M. 1992, *Absent Friend: Coping with the Loss of a Treasured Pet*, Henston Books, High Wycombe, UK.

Leviton, D. 1978, 'The Intimacy/Sexual Needs of the Terminally Ill and Widowed', *Death Education*, vol. 2, pp. 261–80.

Lochner, C. W. & Stevenson, R. G. 1988, 'Music as a Bridge to Wholeness', *Death Studies*, vol. 12, pp. 173–80.

Lyketsos, C. G., Hutton, H., Fishman, M., Schwartz, J., & Treisman, G. J. 1996, 'Psychiatric Morbidity on Entry to an HIV Primary Care Clinic', *AIDS*, vol. 10 no. 9, pp. 1033–9.

McDannell, C. & Lang, B. 1988, *Heaven: A History*, Yale University Press, New Haven.

MacDonald, N. 1993, 'Priorities in Education and Research in Palliative Medicine', *Palliative Medicine*, vol. 7, pp. 65–76.

Mitford, J. 1980, *The American Way of Death*, Quartet Books, London.

Moody, R. A. 1975, *Life after Life*, Bantam, New York.

—— 1993, *Reunions: Visionary Encounters with Departed Loved Ones*, Villard Books, New York.

Moore, V. 1946, *Ho for Heaven! Man's Changing Attitude toward Dying*, E. P. Dutton & Co., New York.

Morris, A. S. (ed.) 1958, *One Thousand Inspirational Things*, Consolidated Book Publishers, Chicago.

Murry, J. M. (ed.) 1983, *Journal of Katherine Mansfield*, The Ecco Press, New York.

National Council for Hospice and Specialist Palliative Care Services 1995, *Specialist Palliative Care: A Statement of Definitions*, Occasional Paper no. 8, National Council for Hospice and Specialist Palliative Care Services, London.

Nettleton, S. & Bunton, R. 1995, 'Sociological Critiques of Health Promotion', in R. Bunton, S. Nettleton, & R. Burrows, *The Sociology of Health Promotion: Critical Analyses of Consumption, Lifestyle and Risk*, Routledge, London, pp. 41–58.

Nichols, K. & Jenkinson, J. 1991, *Leading a Support Group*, Chapman & Hall, London.

Nuland, S. B. 1994, *How We Die*, Chatto & Windus, London.

O'Connor, M. L. & Parker, E. 1995, *Health Promotion: Principles and Practice in the Australian Context*, Allen & Unwin, Sydney.

Osis, K. & Haraldsson, E. 1977, *At the Hour of Our Death*, Avon Books, New York.

'Ottawa Charter for Health Promotion' 1986, *Health Promotion*, vol. 1, pp. iii–v.

Pacholski, R. A. 1986a, 'Death Themes in Music: Resources and Research Opportunities for Death Educators', *Death Studies*, vol. 10, pp. 239–63.

—— 1986b, 'Death Themes in the Visual Arts: Resources and Research Opportunities for Death Educators', *Death Studies*, vol. 10, pp. 59–74.

Parker, J. & Aranda, S. (eds) 1998, *Palliative Care: Explorations and Challenges*, MacLennan & Petty, Sydney.

Parkinson, C. 1979, *The Self-Help Movement in Australia*, Australian Council of Social Service, Sydney.

Pincus, L. 1976, *Death and the Family*, Faber & Faber, London.

Pine, V. 1986, 'The Age of Maturity for Death Education: A Socio-Historical Portrait of the Era 1976–1985', *Death Studies*, vol. 10, pp. 209–31.

Powell, T. J. (ed.) 1990, *Working with Self-Help*, National Association of Social Workers, Silver Spring, Md.

Raphael, B. & Maddison, D. 1972, 'The Family of the Dying Patient', in O. G. Brim, H. E. Freeman, S. Levine, & N. A. Scotch (eds), *The Dying Patient*, Russell Sage, New York, pp. 171–90.

Raudive, K. 1971, *Breakthrough: An Amazing Experiment in Electronic Communication with the Dead*, Colin Smythe, Gerrards Cross, UK.

Reanney, D. 1994, *Music of the Mind: An Adventure into Consciousness*, Hill of Content, Melbourne.

Register, C. 1989, *Living with Chronic Illness: Days of Patience and Passion*, Bantam Books, New York.

Ring, K. 1980, *Life at Death: A Scientific Investigation of the Near-Death Experience*, Coward, McCann & Geoghegan, New York.

Roberts, C. S., Severinsen, C., Carraway, C., Clark, D., Freeman, M., & Daniel, P. 1997, 'Life Changes and Problems Experienced by Young Adults with Cancer', *Journal of Psychosocial Oncology*, vol. 15, no. 1, pp. 15–25.

Rose, G. 1995, *Love's Work*, Chatto & Windus, London.

Ross, H. S. & Mico, P. R. 1980, *Theory and Practice in Health Education*, Mayfield Publishing Company, Palo Alto, Calif.

Rumbold, B. 1998, 'Implications of Mainstreaming Hospice into Palliative Care Services', in J. Parker & S. Aranda (eds), *Palliative Care: Explorations and Challenges*, MacLennan & Petty, Sydney, pp. 3–20.

Saunders, C. 1987, 'What's in a Name?', *Palliative Medicine*, vol. 1, pp. 57–61.

Savary, L. M. & O'Connor, T. J. (eds) 1973, *The Heart Has its Seasons: Reflections on the Human Condition*, Regina Press, New York.

Savary, L. M., O'Connor, T. J., Cullen, R. M., & Plummer, D. M. (eds) 1970, *Listen to Love: Reflections on the Seasons of the Year*, Regina Press, New York.

Schofferman, J. 1988, 'Care of the AIDS Patient', *Death Studies*, vol. 12, pp. 433–49.

Schratz, M. & Walker, R. 1995, *Research as Social Change: New Opportunities for Qualitative Research*, Routledge, London.

Schulz, R., Williamson, G. M., Knapp, J. E., Bookwala, J., Lave, J., & Fello, M. 1995, 'The Psychological, Social, and Economic Impact of Illness among Patients with Recurrent Cancer', *Journal of Psychosocial Oncology*, vol. 13, no. 3, pp. 21–45.

Selby, F. G. (ed.) 1912, *Bacon's Essays*, Macmillan & Co., London.

Sherman, E. & Reid, W. J. (eds) 1994, *Qualitative Research in Social Work*, Columbia University Press, New York.

Sindall, C. 1992, 'Health Promotion and Community Health in Australia', in F. Baum, D. Fry, & I. Lennie (eds), *Community Health: Policy and Practice in Australia*, Pluto Press, Sydney.

Smyth, J. 1986, *A Rationale for Teachers' Critical Pedagogy: A Handbook*, Deakin University Press, Geelong.

Solzhenitsyn, A. 1968, *Cancer Ward*, Penguin Books, Harmondsworth.

Stokols, D. 1992, 'Establishing and Maintaining Healthy Environments: Toward a Social Ecology of Health Promotion', *American Psychologist*, vol. 47, pp. 6–22.

Sussman, M. (ed.) 1985, *Pets and the Family*, Haworth, New York.

Thomas, S. 1992, 'Evaluation Methods in Health Care Programs', in H. Gardner (ed.), *Health Policy: Development, Implementation and Evaluation in Australia*, Longman Cheshire, Melbourne, pp. 73–86.

Thorman, S. 1987, *A Journey through Self Help: An Evaluation of Self Help in Western Australia*, Western Institute of Self Help, Perth.

Tolstoy, L. N. 1960, *The Death of Ivan Ilyich*, Penguin Books, Harmondsworth.

Tones, K., Tilford, S., & Robinson, Y. 1990, *Health Education: Effectiveness and Efficiency*, Chapman & Hall, London.

UNICEF (n.d.), *All for Health: A Resource Book for 'Facts of Life'*, UNICEF, New York.

Vafiadis, P. 1997, *Culture and Attitudes in Palliative Care: Meeting the Needs in General Practice*, report for the General Practice Evaluation Programme, Department of Public Health and Community Medicine, University of Melbourne, Melbourne.

Wacks, V. Q. 1988, 'Educating for Eschatological Concerns of the Older Adult: A Brief Report', *Death Studies*, vol. 12, pp. 329–35.

Wadsworth, Y. 1991, *Everyday Evaluation on the Run*, Action Research Issues Association, Melbourne.

Walter, T. 1997, 'Emotional Reserve and the English Way of Grief', in K. Charmaz, G. Howarth, & A. Kellehear (eds), *The Unknown Country: Death in Australia, Britain, and the USA*, Macmillan, Basingstoke, pp. 127–40.

Wass, A. 1994, *Promoting Health: The Primary Health Care Approach*, W. B. Saunders Balliere Tindall, Sydney.

Waugh, E. 1948, *The Loved One*, Little Brown & Co., Boston.

Weiss, J., Bartsch, H. H., Nagel, G. A., & Unger, C. 1996, 'Psychosocial Care for Cancer Patients: A New Holistic Psychosomatic Approach in Acute Care and Rehabilitation', *Psycho-oncology*, vol. 5, pp. 51–4.

Welch, W. A. 1975, *Talks with the Dead*, Pinnacle Books, New York.

Witzel, L. 1975, 'Behaviour of the Dying Patient', *British Medical Journal*, vol. 2, pp. 81–2.

World Health Organization 1988, *Education for Health: A Manual on Health Education in Primary Health Care*, World Health Organization, Geneva.

—— 1990, *Cancer Pain Relief and Palliative Care*, Technical Report Series no. 804, World Health Organization, Geneva.

Yalom, I. D. 1975, *The Theory and Practice of Group Psychotherapy*, Basic Books, New York.

Zaleski, C. 1987, *Otherworld Journeys: Accounts of Near-Death Experiences in Medieval and Modern Times*, Oxford University Press, New York.

Index